RAW

CHALLENGE

RAW

CHALLENGE

Lisa Montgomery

≫ hatherleigh

))) hatherleigh

Hatherleigh Press is committed to preserving and protecting the natural resources of the earth. Environmentally responsible and sustainable practices are embraced within the company's mission statement.

Visit us at www.hatherleighpress.com and register online for free offers, discounts, special events, and more.

Library of Congress Cataloging-in-Publication Data is available.
ISBN: 978-1-57826-421-6

Cover Design by Carolyn Kasper / DCDesigns
Interior Design by Carolyn Kasper / DCDesigns

Printed in the United States

10 9 8 7 6 5 4 3 2 1

ACKNOWLEDGMENTS

I would like to thank everyone at Kimberton Whole Foods—especially Drew Hunt, who first came up with the idea to hold the Raw Challenge—and all who participated and helped to make Raw Challenge a success. From the challenge itself, to the workshops and the book, none of it would have been possible without the help of the participants (a.k.a. the "Raw Challengers"), Jennifer Vanderslice, and Josh Batman, my rent-a-son. Thank you to everyone who helped to bring the "Raw Challenge" workshop and *Raw Challenge* the book to fruition.

CONTENTS

INTRODUCTION

If you want to transform your life and your health, *Raw Challenge* will help you to do just that. You are about to embark on your own personal Raw Challenge, and using this book as your guide, you will begin the transition to becoming the best "you" you can be. The quest to grow emotionally, spiritually, and physically is a lifelong endeavor. I am always striving to expand and grow beyond my current limitations; in my mind, there is no ceiling on what you can accomplish. Once I started to live a healthier lifestyle with raw foods, I grew so much emotionally and spiritually. You would not believe how much bad food choices and an unhealthy lifestyle can hold you back from reaching your true potential.

Raw Challenge will help you on your journey to transform yourself and your health. To have peace in your heart and mind is a priceless gift. By changing what you eat, you will begin to feel and look better. You'll start to feel better about yourself and your circumstances.

Last fall Drew Hunt, the café manager at Kimberton Whole Foods (my local health food store) approached me about holding a Raw Challenge at their original store in Kimberton, Pennsylvania. As a passionate supporter of the raw lifestyle (not to mention the fact that Kimberton Whole Foods is practically my second home), my response was an immediate, "Sure, let's do it!"

This book is a product of the experiences from this Raw Challenge. The participants in my Challenge were not world renowned raw chefs sequestered to a beautiful desert island—though that would have been nice! The participants, my "Raw Challengers," were real people living in the real world—people you can relate to. They were changing and adapting their lives while balancing their everyday routines at work, at home, with their family and friends. Many of the recipes in this book were created by the Raw Challengers themselves, which means if they can create recipes, so can you. I want you to see that this inspiring group of people is just as amazing as you are, and if they had the courage to change their diet and lifestyle, so can you.

The format that we used for the Raw Challenge is the same format that we have used in this book. We have a proven track record. It worked for our Challengers and it will work for you.

Be content with living and eating a healthy lifestyle. People often think they are giving up what they enjoy by eating healthfully. However, the reality is that when you eat a healthy, raw diet you are actually gaining so much more. One of the biggest benefits of eating raw is that you are emotionally balanced. Not only do you have more energy, but you are also calmer, more at peace. I want to live dynamically, and the only way I have found to do that is to live this lifestyle. Once you change your mind to see what you are gaining you will realize that eating healthy is a wonderfully positive change. Many of us think that the struggle of switching to a healthy diet is going to kill us when in reality *not* eating healthy will kill us. We think if we eat healthy we are sacrificing something, when in reality we are opening a new and exciting world with great and wonderful potential.

> *"What I learned from the Raw Challenge and what I want to share with you is to stay focused on how great you feel. That is the ongoing reward."*
> — DENISE DiJOSEPH (www.MiAura.com)

Whether you are a novice or have been eating a raw diet for years, we all have our own reasons for choosing raw foods. As baby boomers, many of us thought that we somehow would be exempt from aging and getting wrinkles. Yet we were wrong, and the wrinkles came. The good news is, by living and eating healthy, I honestly feel as if I am getting younger instead of older. In fact, my general practitioner once said to me that I am the healthiest person in his practice, which sees approximately 3,500 patients. If you eat healthfully, and get regular exercise and rest, chances are you will no longer need to see your doctor other than for annual checkups. In addition to improving your overall health, a raw diet can also increase your energy levels. I have found that I now have so much energy that I leave the Energizer Bunny® in the dust. I always strive to be the best that I can be and to feel my best, and eating raw enables me to continue this quest.

Perhaps you are not switching to raw foods for health reasons, but because you want to look good. When you start to eat healthfully, your body feels better and it shows on your face. There is a "raw glow" on the skin of those who eat healthy. I have had more people say to me, "You know why people will want to eat like you: because of your skin." I also know people who, after starting a raw diet, notice that their grey hair has turned back to their original hair color.

"My adventure into raw food began in October, 2009. Surprisingly, I discovered JOY in the most unexpected place. What started as an exploration into healing resulted in a whole new toolbox for creating food that is literally ALIVE with color, texture, flavor, healing nutrients and LIFE! I quickly fell in love with a whole new palette of ingredients . . . and a new palate for tasting them.

Raw is beautiful. It's alive . . . and it offers me an incredible challenge to CREATE new and exciting textures that are decadent, delicious and nutritious. And the best is, I'm eating food that is chock full of healing properties, the way nature intended. Uncooked food from nature comes with its own enzymes, which means the body does not have to work as hard to digest it. If you are chronically ill, this enables your body to conserve some of its resources that can be used towards healing."

— BARBARA SHEVKUN of Rawfully Tempting
(www.rawfullytempting.com)

Healthy eating will not only strengthen you physically but it will also give you an opportunity to be strengthened emotionally and spiritually. Eating and living healthy empowers you and gives you confidence in what you think and feel in the here and now. When living a healthy lifestyle you are no longer numbing yourself with cooked foods, meat, alcohol, and so on. This gives you an opportunity to really look inward and decide whether you like what you see or if you need to make some changes in your diet and in your life. Oftentimes, we spend too much of our lives living in a fog, without being fully awake and living in the present. The raw lifestyle gives you an opportunity to truly wake up.

HOW TO FOLLOW THE RAW CHALLENGE

We've broken this book down into three main sections to make it easier for you to read and incorporate into your lifestyle. In Part I, you will find an overview of what a raw diet entails, along with a discussion of the many health benefits of a raw diet. You will also find guidance on what you can expect during and after your Raw Challenge, based on the real-life experiences of myself and my Raw Challengers. Throughout the book, we have also included helpful tips and tricks to help you on this journey.

Part II makes you feel like I am right there with you holding your hand throughout your personal journey. You will find entries for each of the 30 days in your Raw Challenge. Each day comes complete with meal suggestions for Breakfast, Lunch, and Dinner, using the recipes found in Part III. You can also select a daily snack from Part III to keep you full and satisfied all day long. The daily entries in Part II also include helpful tips as well as inspirational quotes and testimonials from fellow Raw Challengers to keep you motivated. Each day also includes journaling space for you to add your own notes and experiences.

Part III offers over 75 wonderful recipes from Kimberton Whole Foods, my Raw Challengers, and even some from my own personal collection. We hope you enjoy trying our recipes as much as we enjoyed creating them. Also, don't be afraid to try creating some of your own recipes! If you are new to raw foods, start by trying out some of the dishes in Part III. Once you feel comfortable making raw meals, let your creativity run wild and put together your own raw creations!

As you may know from some of my previous books, such as *Raw Inspiration*, I really enjoy using quotes, sayings, and stories that inspire me in my daily journey. Similarly, I have included wonderful testimonials from each of the Raw Challengers who wished to share their stories. These stories will touch your heart and quite possibly move you to tears, as they did me. Turn to these stories any time you are in need of some motivation or encouragement throughout your own personal Raw Challenge.

The Raw Challenge, and all of its facets, has the opportunity to touch and transform every part of you. How do I know this? Because I live this lifestyle and I have seen it happen to myself and many others. So please join me on this journey toward becoming the new and improved *you*.

> *"I love a challenge. So when Lisa decided to have her raw food challenge, I was psyched! Sharing a journey with like-minded people toward a common goal is fun and inspiring. I knew I would be more likely to stay committed when there were other people who expected me to do the best I could do, and report back on what I had actually done. For me, that was a great way to share this particular journey."*
>
> —DAWN LIGHT

PART I:
WHY RAW FOOD?

As you embark on this Raw Challenge, you may encounter friends and family that ask why you are following a raw diet. As was mentioned in the Introduction, there are many benefits to the raw lifestyle, but you will come to find that we each have our own personal reasons for making the switch. When I attended the Institute of Integrative Nutrition (IIN) in New York, New York several years ago to become certified as a Holistic Healthcare Practitioner, my diet was already predominantly raw. During my studies at IIN we were introduced to many different eating styles including South Beach, Aravic, Atkins, and, of course, raw. Although my diet was predominantly raw, I chose to eat the way we were being taught at the time. So if we were being taught Atkins, I would eat an Atkins diet. If we were being taught microbiotic, I would eat a microbiotic diet. However, I soon came to realize that these eating styles were *diets*, not lifestyles. The raw diet is a raw lifestyle. When I tried the other diets they made me physically sick. On the other hand, the raw lifestyle resonates down to my soul. When I eat this way I feel at peace, which is a gift that no money can buy. Once you begin to feel that peace in your heart and notice how your body works for you on a daily basis, you will come to understand the answer to the question, "why raw foods?"

Raw foods include fruits, vegetables, nuts, grains, and seeds that are uncooked. Because raw foods are never heated above 118°F, they retain all of their nutrients, allowing your body to get the most out of your food.

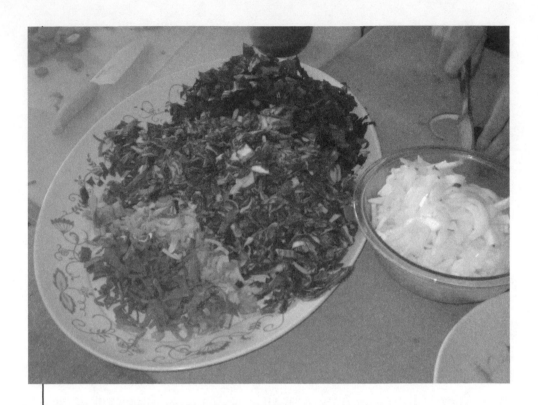

While a raw diet is a lifestyle change, it's much easier to follow than you may think. For me, a typical day starts with juicing wheatgrass in my Tribest Green Star juicer. Sometimes I also make a vegetable juice in my juicer and store it in a glass jar to drink throughout the day. For breakfast I also have a smoothie which I make in my Vitamix® high-speed blender. Lunch usually consists of a salad of greens, sprouts, fermented sauerkraut, chopped vegetables, and a pâté. Many times, I don't even eat dinner as I find that I'm not hungry. Instead, I usually have a vegetable juice or watermelon juice in place of dinner. If I do feel like I need more than just a drink, I will have a handful of almonds or a few

raw crackers. As you can see, my raw diet is really very simple and very basic
. . . and yours can be, too!

WHAT TO EXPECT FROM THE RAW CHALLENGE

Now that you know what it means to follow a raw diet, let's go over what you can expect to experience during your own Raw Challenge.

At the start of the first meeting for our Raw Challenge, I asked each of the participants to go around the room to introduce themselves and share what brought them to the Challenge. Some people were facing a health crisis and needed to make changes fast; some were already in the midst of changing their lifestyle and needed to take it to another level, while others just needed a refresher on following a raw diet. The great thing about the Raw Challenge is that, no matter where you are in your journey, you can tailor the program to your own needs. Using the meal suggestions in Part II, along with the recipes in Part III, you can create a program that fits your unique needs and preferences, which makes the Raw Challenge even more fun and exciting!

When you first embark on your Raw Challenge, changing your diet may feel scary and uncertain, which is why it can be helpful to start with something easy. Participants in my Raw Challenge were everyday people, not professional raw chefs, so we had to make this Challenge easy to follow in the real world. In order to do this, I made sure to start things off simple by making smoothies.

During the first week in your transition to a raw diet, you are bound to be nervous. You may be asking yourself, How will my body feel? Will I still be hungry? What should I expect? The first thing you will need to get used to is that when you eat raw you will feel light and refreshed in your stomach rather than feeling stuffed and heavy. Once you get used to the fact that you won't starve to death without that full feeling, you can start to enjoy the experiences that will begin almost immediately. Some of my Raw Challengers immediately noticed they slept better, they had more energy, and their skin glowed. One thing that may happen when you change your diet is a detox effect. Detoxification did not happen immediately for me, but when it did, it felt like I had a cold. Detox is a result of your body trying to get rid of everything that has built up from poor eating habits. Your body is so happy that you are now taking care of yourself, and it wants to rid itself of the junk. But you can't get rid of it fast enough, so you can end up with flu-like symptoms and sometimes even rashes. Although detox can be tough, it is only temporary and is a good sign that your body is responding to the healthy changes you are making in your diet. Stick with it, and your body will thank you by the end of your Raw Challenge.

When starting your Challenge, you should also assess whether you want to transition gradually into a raw diet or dive right in. Some people go cold turkey while others choose to do it gradually. Your personality and body type will determine which is best for you. Whatever you choose, remember to be gentle to yourself and to your body.

You may also find that you don't need to eat nearly as much as you used to in order to feel full. The first time people come to my raw potlucks they are blown away at how beautiful everything looks and smells. They fill up their plate and are then amazed by how wonderful and alive everything tastes. Finally, after only a few mouthfuls they are filled. When you eat raw foods you are eating live food and are receiving all the nourishment from the food, which is why you get filled up so quickly. When you eat food cooked over 118°F all the nutritional value has been cooked out of the food and you have to keep eating until you feel full or satiated (or both). People often assume that eating raw is expensive, but what they don't realize is that they will end up eating a fraction of what they used to, so they end up saving money. Plus you will also save money by being healthy and not spending money on doctor bills.

> *"It's hard in the beginning but aside from quitting smoking and learning to properly and regularly practice meditation, I can think of nothing that has improved my health and life so much a raw vegan diet."*
>
> —DREW HUNT

The amazing gift of this lifestyle is that you start showing results almost immediately, so by the time you reach the second week you should already start to see significant changes. By now your body is starting to adjust to your new diet and lifestyle. If you have experienced detox symptoms, they should begin to subside now, but keep in mind that everyone's body is different and reacts differently. After those challenges have faded it just gets better. You will start to feel better and look better. What more can you ask for?

I was so excited for the Challengers at the midway point of their Raw Challenge. The results they were having after a short period of time were phenomenal. They came into the workshop chattering like long lost buddies and everyone could hardly wait to share their results. Even those who experienced some detoxification were still happy that they were moving forward. They were excited that they could create recipes from everyday ingredients and they loved incorporating ingredients, like young Thai coconut, which they would have never even attempted before. By the midway point, the Challengers had also lost weight, which they were ecstatic about.

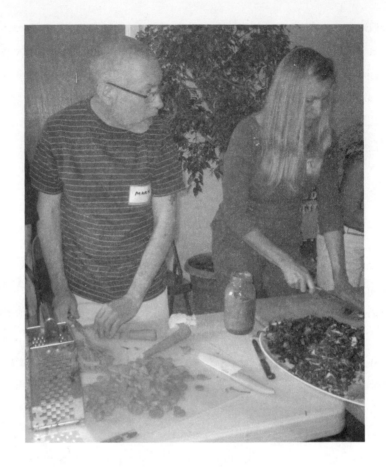

Photo courtesy of Tammy Jerome

Toward the end of your Raw Challenge, you should start to become more comfortable with your new, healthy diet. Eating raw foods will feel more like second-nature and you may even try your hand at inventing your very own raw recipes! For the final meeting of my Raw Challenge, I had all of the Challengers bring their favorite raw dish. The cool thing was, for some this was their first raw potluck, and they all did an amazing job in creating their own recipes. If you are doing your Challenge as a group, try holding your own raw potluck to share recipes and swap stories about your experiences. This is a great way to connect with your fellow Challengers and assess your progress over the 30 days.

TRANSITIONING TO RAW FOODS
By Irene Bojczuk

Irene Bojczuk, one of our Raw Challengers, provided an easy-to-follow way to transition to raw foods. I couldn't have said it better myself, and Irene has graciously allowed me to share this with you in the hopes that it will help you to make the transition to a healthier way of living. Many people *want* to eat and live healthier—they just don't know where to begin. These guidelines can help ease you into the transition.

STAGE 1
Quit alcohol, quit smoking and quit any recreational drugs.

Have a fruit smoothie for breakfast. Include enough greens so that it still tastes fruity and delicious (over time you can work your way up to adding more greens).

STAGE 2
Make sure you get 8½ to 9 hours of sleep each night, especially as you do these transitions. Nothing else repairs the body better than good quality rest. If you wake up naturally, ready to get out of bed, you know you're truly rested.

STAGE 3

Replace all refined sugar products with fruit. If you're craving sugar it's because you haven't had enough fruit earlier in the day (the glucose in fruit is what your muscles really need for energy).

Replace all junk food with crunchy raw vegetables like celery, red and orange peppers, or asparagus. The minerals in these vegetables will eventually handle your cravings.

Replace all soda and carbonation with water, not bottled juices.

STAGE 4

Eliminate all dairy—including milk, cheeses, butter, and whey—often found in protein powders and many refined foods.

Eliminate all meat—red, white, boiled, or raw. Meat requires more digestive enzymes than we naturally have and the body will steal calcium from your bones to buffer the acid found in meat.

Reduce or eliminate all coffee and all caffeinated beverages (you may take it in stages if you're really addicted).

Start eating more raw and less cooked food. Start by trying sprouted lentils and see if they agree with you. When still cooking, lightly steam your food rather than boiling, sautéing, or baking.

STAGE 5

Eliminate all grains and grain-based products. Start by removing all wheat and glutens first, followed by corn, and eventually all grains.

STAGE 6

Eliminate legumes such as lentils, lima beans, and kidney beans. Especially (and most importantly) eliminate all soybeans and soy products of every kind—tofu, edamame, soy sauce, tamari, etc.

> *Note from Lisa: There are many raw foodists who do soak beans and lentils, and sprout them to include in salads or pâtés.*

STAGE 7

By now you are eating only raw fruits, vegetables, nuts, greens, and seeds and are sleeping until fully rested. You are eating fruits and greens as smoothies or whole for breakfast and lunch. You are using a minimal amount of nuts, avocados, and seeds as well as seed and nut butters.

IMPORTANT: Find out how many calories your body needs daily to function by using this formula:

Ideal Weight x 100 = Base Calorie Need + Amount of Calories Used
by Your Activity Level

Make sure you are getting enough calories in the right proportions (80% carbohydrates, 10% fats, 10% proteins). This is a major key in being able to succeed. Not getting enough calories is a common reason for cravings and indulgences.

> *Note from Lisa: Here, Irene follows Dr. Doug Graham's 80/10/10 proportions. This is a great guideline, but you may need to tweak the*

percentages for your body and its needs. In the past I've tried being very strict with the 80/10/10 and found I needed more fat in my diet.

STAGE 8

Practice fitness activities every day to build muscle and exercise aerobically to raise your heart rate.

Get some fresh air and sunshine every day, for at least 15 minutes. Indoor air is not as supportive as fresh air.

STAGE 9

You have by this time most certainly eliminated the need for any supplements and powders.

In the case of medications, reduce them carefully by consulting with your physician.

> *Note from Lisa: Because of the quality of today's food, we can't always get everything we need. Depending on the state of your health at the outset, you may still want to take some supplements to support your body's needs as necessary.*

STAGE 10

Set a goal to reduce your body fat percentage. A lower percentage of body fat enables optimal bodily functions for absorbing and utilizing hydration, releasing toxins, and many more.

TIPS AND TRICKS

In the following section you will find several tips to set you up for success before embarking on your Raw Challenge. For additional guidance, you can also refer to any of the wonderful books and websites in the Resources section on page 217.

An easy way to help you transition into a healthy lifestyle is to drink more water. I drink water all day. Many times we feel tired or hungry, but all we really need to do is drink water. Drink water first and then decide whether you need to eat. Since your body is mostly made up of water you need to keep replenishing the water all the time. Drinking water helps to cleanse your system as well, which means when you are detoxifying the water will help to flush out the toxins from your body. Replace sodas and coffees with water, vegetable juice, and fruit juices. By making your own juices you not only get to be creative but the juices you create will be fresh and free of any preservatives. Remember, fresh is always best.

Be sure to get plenty of rest. You are making big changes to your body and rest is healing. Also there are statistics that say if you want to lose weight you need to get at least 8 hours of sleep each night.

Check with a doctor if you have any medical conditions. If you already have any health concerns like diabetes, be sure to consult with your doctor and explain that you are radically changing your diet. Together, you can come up with a raw diet plan that will work safely for you.

TAKE A DEEP BREATH

I was speaking recently with a friend on the topic of breathing. She said, "I used to breathe so I wouldn't die." And I said, "Now you breathe to live." This is the power of the healing breath. People use this deep breath technique in meditation. Most people breathe shallowly. It is much healthier for you emotionally, spiritually, and physically to breath deeper. When my Mom was having congestive heart failure, her cardiologist told her to practice deep breathing to help calm her down and ease her stress. When you breathe deeply, there's a real feeling of peace. You're releasing tension and strengthening your heart, mind, and soul. It's one of the best, easiest changes you can make to feel better!

Don't be afraid to experiment. When I first started eating and drinking raw, I always followed recipes precisely because I was accustomed to traditional cooking methods. However, most raw chefs and teachers simply throw in ingredients without measuring. After a while, you just innately know or learn what goes well together, what you like, and how much spice a dish will need. Raw un-cooking is more forgiving, unlike traditional cooking where, if you do not follow the recipe precisely, the dish can be ruined. Once you become more comfortable with raw recipes, you can experiment with throwing together new dishes based on what you have available and what you are in the mood for. With raw foods, it almost always comes out tasting really good, and if you don't quite like the taste, you can always add a pinch of this or a dollop of that.

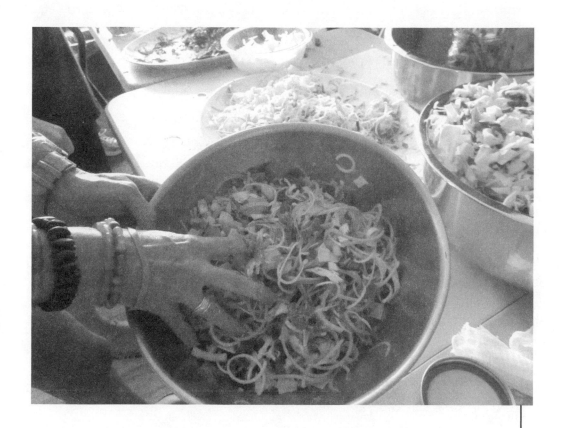

Juicing your fruits and vegetables can provide your body with much-needed nutrients in a tasty and convenient form. If you don't have time to make your own juices, you can turn to healthy juice bars and restaurants. However, if you want to make your own juices at home, it's best to use a juicer. Believe it or not, I have five different juicers (Walker, Omega, Champion, Jack LaLane™, and Tribest), but my favorite has been the Tribest Green Star juicer, because it does everything. When you juice fruits and vegetables, you can also add assorted supplements to kick the drink up a notch. Here are a few examples:

- Aloe vera: 100 percent pure digestive healer
- Bee pollen: promotes vitality and stamina
- Cayenne: revitalizes the respiratory system
- Vitamin C: strengthens the immune system
- Flaxseed oil: benefits the cardiovascular system
- Ginger: relieves nausea and indigestion
- Raw honey: contains healthful minerals, vitamins, carbohydrates, and enzymes
- Spirulina: boosts energy and supports cellular health
- Protein powder: helps to burn fat and build muscle
- Complete meal powder: plant-based protein that contains every nutrient necessary for optimum health (I use this every day in my smoothie)

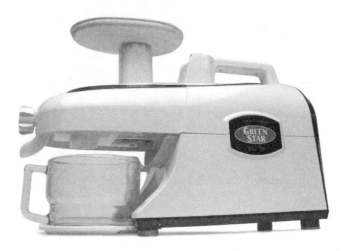

Photo courtesy of Tribest (www.tribest.com)

TIPS FOR JUICING

When juicing, place the fine screen over the twin gears. Then attach the pulp discharge casing to the outlet, adjusting the knob in place, and loosen the knob as you juice to allow the pulp to come out (when I juice wheatgrass, I do not use the knob, at all). Place the pitcher under the juice outlet to catch the juice, and keep a bowl or bag under the pulp discharge outlet to catch the pulp. Remember to save your pulp, as you can use it in crackers and burgers or even feed it to your pets.

If you juice nothing else, I strongly urge you to start your day by juicing wheatgrass. It is full of vitamins and minerals, which makes it cleansing, healing, and detoxifying. Wheatgrass is a stand-alone juice. I start almost every day by juicing several ounces. I do not combine wheatgrass with anything else. It is also best to drink on an empty stomach. Remember: you should not drink wheatgrass quickly. Instead, sip and swish a mouthful at a time. Wheatgrass is available pre-cut and packaged, or can be bought uncut on a mat, which is typically a more economical option. To cut wheatgrass from the mat, use either a straight edge blade or a sharp knife or shears. Place the wheatgrass in a large re-sealable bag with paper towels to soak up the moisture and store it in your refrigerator. I start my day by juicing the wheatgrass in my Tribest Green Star Elite juicer. I also put the wheatgrass mat out on my picnic table in the warm weather months to produce a second growth. It won't be quite as potent as the first cutting, but it is still beneficial to one's health. It's a great way to kick start your health in a positive direction.

> *"Like most people, I usually crave something sweet at the end of my meal (especially after dinner). Instead of going for that cookie or piece of chocolate, I'll pop a couple raw cacao nips into my mouth. The bitterness immediately cuts my craving for sweetness, the deep richness sates my want for dark chocolate, and best of all, the cacao is actually really good for me."*
>
> — KEN ALAN, Concierge, Food & Travel Writer

Using frozen fruits: Be careful when purchasing frozen fruit as it may contain added refined sugar or preservatives, which will defeat the purpose of trying to eat and live a healthy lifestyle. The best way to make sure that there are no preservatives or sugar in your frozen fruit is to freeze it yourself. When my fruit comes in, I use it as well as freeze it. When organic fruit is on sale at my local market, I will also buy several cases and freeze them so I can pull them out when I need them.

Watermelon juice: Watermelon, besides tasting wonderful, is also a natural diuretic and is a great option for transitioning to a raw diet because it is a food that many people are familiar with. I even know some healing centers who serve their patients watermelon juice because of the healing properties. I make watermelon juice because it tastes great, and I drink it year-round. My favorite time of the day to drink watermelon juice is in the evening after I exercise or when I'm feeling dehydrated. The watermelon juice helps me feel satiated. In the evening when you might have a sweet tooth, drinking a glass of watermelon juice fills you up and takes care of the sweet tooth. We've all heard not to eat after sundown or three hours before you go to bed to give your body time to digest before going to sleep. Watermelon juice is one raw food that you can have after sundown because it will digest easily. To make watermelon juice, you simply cut the fruit off the rind, place it in your Vitamix® high-speed blender, and blend. The fruit turns into juice very rapidly.

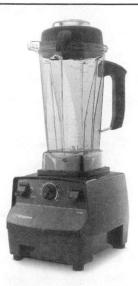

Reproduced and reprinted with the permission of
Vita-Mix Corporation (www.vitamix.com)

HIGH-SPEED BLENDERS

There are several high-speed-powered blenders out there, but my favorite is the Vitamix® blender. The Vitamix® high-speed blender has the speed and power to blend nuts, seeds, and ice quickly. If you attempt to make nut pates (or even simply juice a watermelon) in a regular blender, it just does not have the power or speed to do the job like the Vitamix® blender does. While a juicer and high-speed-powered blender are certainly investments, the good news is you will use them daily, and they will most likely last for the rest of your life. They will be worth every penny that you spend on them once you begin to enjoy your transformation to a healthy, raw diet.

Watercress: Watercress, like mustard greens, is a cruciferous vegetable and, like its cousins broccoli and cabbage, has been recognized as an important source of calcium, iron, and folic acid. Perhaps the best incentive to add this delicious green to your culinary repertoire is the exciting research that came out of the University of Ulster (United Kingdom) about the anti-cancer properties of watercress. This study found that daily intake of watercress can significantly reduce an important cancer trigger; namely DNA damage to white blood cells. Eating watercress salad has also been shown to lower cholesterol and improve absorption of lutein and beta-carotene, which are key minerals for eye health and the prevention of age-related conditions such as cataracts. When eaten raw, watercress is prized for its peppery flavor. You can also mix watercress with fruit for a variety of flavor sensations.

Sundried tomatoes: I make my own sundried tomatoes in my Tribest Sedona dehydrator. When my tomatoes come in season, one of the ways that I harvest them, besides popping them in my mouth, is to slice them thinly, place on the racks of my Tribest Sedona dehydrator, and dehydrate them until dry. I store the tomatoes in air-tight, zip-lock bags. When using vacuum-seal bags,

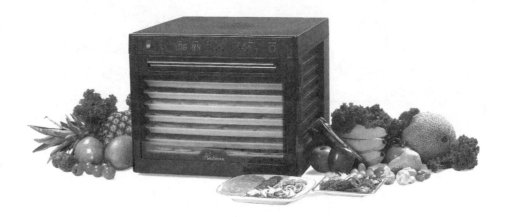

Photo courtesy of Tribest (www.tribest.com)

I actually double bag them. If you do not, the bugs can eat through the bags. They like the tomatoes, too. I am selfish: I do not want to share with the bugs.

ORGANIZING YOUR OWN RAW CHALLENGE

The easiest way to organize a Raw Challenge is to start with your family, friends, and co-workers. Let them know you are starting a Raw Challenge and ask if they would like to participate. For an even larger group, encourage them to bring their friends. Everyone loves food and getting together; now you can all get together and feel better, too!

Set a date, time, and meeting place for the Raw Challenge. Send out an email or newsletter, or post it on Facebook to let everyone know the particulars.

On the day of your first meeting, be sure to come prepared with a plan on what you want to discuss and what dishes you want to share with the group. In my case, I knew there were certain dishes, raw food preparation techniques, and general facts that I wanted to share to help the Raw Challengers begin to incorporate these challenges into their daily lives. The goal is to make it simple, there is no need to overcomplicate anything.

An easy way to start your group's Raw Challenge is to simply use the guidelines in this book. Start by finding out exactly where everyone in the group is at: what their goals and objectives are. You will also want to find out how much they know about this lifestyle. These details will provide you with a starting point. If they know nothing about raw foods you will need to educate them on the basics—what's raw, what's not, how to prepare, and how to succeed. Feel free to demonstrate some sample dishes—I had a lot of success that way. Always keep it simple. If you overcomplicate the demos or the challenge, no one will stick with it. Instead they will go home feeling confused or overwhelmed.

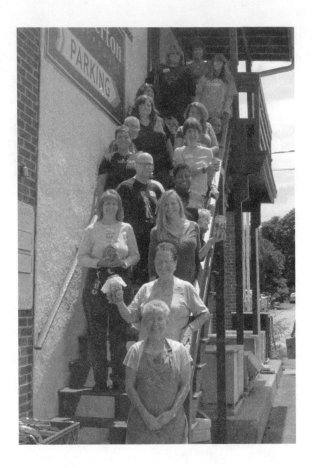

My Raw Challengers and I met once a week during our challenge. This gives you the chance to check in with the needs of your participants and see how they're doing. For our "Finish Line" celebration, we had a raw potluck where each challenger brought a raw dish they had created and prepared. It was a great way to share the new ingredients and techniques with the other participants. Plus, if someone had never tried a certain dish or technique, they could learn from the experiences of their co-Challengers. In the end, the best advice I can give is to just learn by doing, and have fun doing it!

PART II:

THE 30-DAY RAW CHALLENGE COMPANION

DAY 1

Recipes

Breakfast: Neapolitan Smoothie (see page 82)

Lunch: Outstanding Miso Sesame Dressing & Kale Salad (see page 118)

Dinner: Smokey Backyard Tomato Soup with Hot Red Pepper Sauce (see page 123)

Daily Fact

You can juice just about any soft fruits or vegetables, and certain foods such as wheatgrass need to be juiced in order to break down the fiber and cellulose, making digestion much easier.

Daily Affirmation

"The trouble with always trying to preserve the health of the body is that it is so difficult to do without destroying the health of the mind."

—G.K. Chesterton

Challenger Notes / Log Entries

DAY 2

Recipes

Breakfast: Young Thai Coconut Smoothie (see page 66)

Lunch: Thai Tomato Salad (see page 119)

Dinner: Raw Vegetable Pasta (see page 125)

Daily Fact

When your diet consists of more than 75% raw foods, here are just some of the improvements likely to happen to you:

- More energy
- Up to 3 hours less sleep needed
- Weight loss
- Clarity of mind and better memory
- More beautiful skin
- Improved immune system
- Improved fertility
- Prevent or even reverse diabetes

Daily Affirmation

"Did you ever stop to taste a carrot? Not just eat it, but taste it? You can't taste the beauty and energy of the earth in a Twinkie."

— ASTRID ALAUDA

Challenger Notes / Log Entries

_____

_____

_____

_____

_____

_____

_____

_____

DAY 3

Recipes
Breakfast: Water-Based Smoothie (see page 67)

Lunch: Stuffed Peppers (see page 120)

Dinner: Baby Bella Burgers (see page 128)

Daily Fact
Raw foodists choose food that is not processed, sprayed with herbicides, pesticides and that is not genetically modified. If you eat raw you contribute to a cleaner world.

Daily Affirmation
"By cleansing your body on a regular basis and eliminating as many toxins as possible from your environment, your body can begin to heal itself, prevent disease, and become stronger and more resilient than you ever dreamed possible!"

　　—DR. EDWARD GROUP III, founder of the Global Healing Center

. . . From Real Raw Challengers
This challenge seemed easy at first, but I was wrong. I had a fruit smoothie in the morning with an apple, then I would have a salad for lunch, and chicken with a garden salad for dinner. On the second day I had a headache. But it went by quick. From eating a ton of fruits and vegetables, I had a lot of energy. At the end of the first week I lost 4 pounds! I kept up the good work for the second week and lost 3 pounds. When the challenge was over I was so glad: I had lost 7 pounds!"

　　—ALLISON JEROME

Challenger Notes / Log Entries

DAY 4

Recipes
Breakfast: Tammy's Breakfast Smoothie (see page 68)

Lunch: Root Salad (see page 106)

Dinner: Healing Soup (see page 132)

Daily Fact
It's a misconception that you can only eat cold foods when you're on a raw food diet. You can eat warm foods, just don't heat them above 120°F (water 160°F). Most people cook their food and then let it cool off until about 110°F before they eat it anyway.

Daily Affirmation
"The health of people is really the foundation upon which all their happiness and all their power as a state depend."

—BENJAMIN DISRAELI

Challenger Notes / Log Entries

_____

_____

_____

_____

_____

_____

_____

_____

_____

_____

DAY 5

Recipes

Breakfast: Karen's Morning Snacks (see page 69)

Lunch: Tammy's Fruit Salad (see page 92)

Dinner: I Can't Believe This Isn't Pasta (see page 126)

Daily Fact

Meat is not necessarily excluded from a raw food diet. There is evidence suggesting a raw vegan diet supplemented by small amounts of meat and/or fish gives you the optimum balance of nutritional requirements. Think Sashimi as part of your raw food journey!

Daily Affirmation

"We can eliminate heart disease, cancer, diabetes, and weight problems. Go back to the basic foods, become vegetarian and then go vegan, raw. And you'll understand what we're talking about."

—LINDA BLAIR, ACTRESS

. . . From Real Raw Challengers

"In 3 months, I lost a total of 35 lbs. During this time, my insulin was decreased from 18 units daily to 10 units, then to 8 units, 6 units, 4 units, 2 units, then ZERO units daily. I am looking forward to my next appointment with my doctor, as I'm hoping to hear that I will be able to discontinue my oral Type 2 Diabetes medication as well."

—ROBERT CHARLES WHITE, PH.D

Challenger Notes / Log Entries

_____

_____

_____

_____

DAY 6

Recipes
Breakfast: Granny Granola (see page 70)

Lunch: Sprout Salad (see page 93)

Dinner: Trine's Seed Burgers (see page 133)

Daily Fact
Many raw foodists are tempted to focus primarily on including fruits in their diet, and who can blame them? In many cases fruits are sweeter, and their natural sugars can provide a quick pick-me-up late in the day. But it is important to remember that, nutritionally speaking, the green vegetables are going to give you more bang for your buck every time, with more nutrients from less plant matter. The key, as in all things, lies in the happy balance between the two.

Daily Affirmation
"A man too busy to take care of his health is like a mechanic too busy to take care of his tools."

—Spanish Proverb

Challenger Notes / Log Entries

_____

_____

_____

_____

_____

_____

_____

_____

DAY 7

Recipes
Breakfast: Nuts about Granola (see page 71)

Lunch: Spicy Tropical Jicama Salsa & Salad (see page 100)

Dinner: Mock Chicken Salad (see page 129)

Daily Fact
Organic, raw flaxseed is high in Omega 3. The human body cannot produce Omega 3 fatty acids, which are an essential part of the human diet. Most commonly found in fish and eggs, good raw food alternatives are ground flaxseeds, walnuts and pumpkin seeds.

Daily Affirmation
"It is significant to note that those who live on vegetarian food are less prone to diseases, whereas non-vegetarians are subject to more diseases. Why? Because animal food is incompatible with the needs of the human body."

—SRI SATHYA SAI BABA, Indian spiritual leader

Challenger Notes / Log Entries

_____

_____

_____

_____

_____

_____

_____

_____

DAY 8

Recipes
Breakfast: Raw Banana Pancakes (see page 72)

Lunch: Creamy Beet and Horseradish Dip & Horseradish & Dill Crackers (see page 98)

Dinner: Happy Harvest Salad (see page 109)

Daily Fact
You don't necessarily have to give up bread, cakes, or cookies. There are real "raw" alternatives to many cooked foods. A *dehydrator* is a food processor which "slow cooks" at a temperature of less than 120°F, the temperature at which "living" enzymes in food are destroyed.

Daily Affirmation
"Nothing will benefit human health and increase chances for survival of life on Earth as much as the evolution to a vegetarian diet."

—ALBERT EINSTEIN

. . . From Real Raw Challengers
"Honestly, this change in attitude—basically, taking the standpoint that if my ancestors didn't eat it or if I couldn't get it locally, then I wouldn't eat it—made all the difference, as well as an understanding of nutrient density versus eating to be full. Since I've been eating this lifestyle, my health has been tremendous, as has been my wife's."

—SCOTT GRYZBECK

Challenger Notes / Log Entries

_____

_____

_____

DAY 9

Recipes
Breakfast: Fresh Fruit Salad with Macadamia Cream (see page 73)
Lunch: Creamy Cucumber Soup (see page 121)
Dinner: Sun Burgers (see page 135)

Daily Fact
Coconut water is one of the purest forms of waters. With no cholesterol, more electrolytes than any fruit or vegetable, and enough vitamin C to meet the body's daily needs, it is one of the most naturally nutritious drinks. In addition, coconut water also contains trace amounts of copper, phosphorous, and sulfur, making it an excellent supplement for correcting electrolyte imbalance. Fat-free, low in carbohydrates and calories, coconut water's nutrition factor also shows that it contains many elements of the vitamin B group. Coconut water helps maintain body temperature and natural fluid levels and helps carry vital nutrients and oxygen throughout the body.

Daily Affirmation
"To my mind, the life of a lamb is no less precious than that of a human being. I should be unwilling to take the life of a lamb for the sake of the human body."
—MOHANDAS GANDHI

Challenger Notes / Log Entries

_____

_____

_____

_____

_____

DAY 10

Recipes

Breakfast: Lisa's Every Day Green Drink (see page 74)

Lunch: Fermented Italian Green Beans (see page 117)

Dinner: Popeye Would Be Jealous Crackers & Sunflower Pâté (see page 101)

Daily Fact

A study of over 500 raw volunteers concluded that people who have been on a raw foods diet for two years or more experienced significant improvements on many emotional, mental, and spiritual levels.

Daily Affirmation

"Obesity is nothing more than backed-up cooked-food waste trapped in the body. No amount of raw plant food is fattening, only cooked food is fattening. Eating raw bankrupts all the complex theories as to why and how people become fat."

—ARLIN, DINI & WOLFE, *Nature's First Law: The Raw-Food Diet* (Maul Bros. Publishing, San Diego, CA, 1998)

. . . From Real Raw Challengers

"I have been on a natural healing path for the past 30 years. Eventually my journey culminated in the raw foods arena which brought dramatic changes in my health such as greater mental clarity, a huge increase of energy, clear skin, and a true glow of health."

—SHERYLL CHAVARRIA

Challenger Notes / Log Entries

DAY 11

Recipes
Breakfast: Vanilla Crème Smoothie (see page 75)

Lunch: Stuffed Peppers (see page 120)

Dinner: Chilled Cucumber Mint Soup (see page 107)

Daily Fact
One of the major benefits of a raw food diet is that it is alkaline-forming, as opposed to the acid-forming content of the SAD (Standard American Diet). But many brands of bottled water are so heavily steamed and filtered that all mineral content is removed, leaving the water slightly acidic! The solution? Filter your water from your own tap to remove contaminants while retaining all the important mineral content to keep your water live and raw!

Daily Affirmation
"To a great extent, when you take up the raw food diet, you become a new and different and better person. You don't just stay the old person, only a little healthier. . . You become more of your essence, your true and natural self. You become a person who is more a part of the one great life of Nature and less of the confused human world."

—JOE ALEXANDER, *Blatant Raw Foodist Propaganda!*

Challenger Notes / Log Entries

_____

_____

_____

_____

_____

_____

DAY 12

Recipes
Breakfast: Almond Milk Smoothie (see page 63)

Lunch: Thai Tomato Salad (see page 119)

Dinner: Italian Eggplant Chips & Almond Hummus (see page 103)

Daily Fact
Discover bee pollen! Bee pollen contains more than 96 different nutrients, including every single nutrient that you need to live. It's made up of 40% protein. It's a natural energizer, slows down the aging process, and lowers cholesterol levels. It alleviates allergies, improves endurance, strength and mental clarity. It also promotes weight loss: the rate at which your body burns fat, and it reduces cravings.

Daily Affirmation
"It was tough at first because cooked food is addictive . . . Once I cleansed my body of the cooked-food residues, I no longer craved cooked food. What a liberating experience!"

—STEPHEN ARLIN, *Raw Power, Building Strength & Muscle Naturally* (Maul Bros. Publ., San Diego, CA, 1998)

. . . From Real Raw Challengers
"During this challenge, I found out about myself. One self discovery was that I am a carb/junk food addict. When I am stressed I crave carbs and sugars. As a recovering addict, I needed to find something else to eat or do when I am stressed. I needed to change the word raw food DIET into LIFESTYLE."

—LU ANN

Challenger Notes / Log Entries

_____

_____

_____

DAY 13

Recipes

Breakfast: Raw Banana Pancakes (see page 72)

Lunch: Happy Harvest Salad (see page 109)

Dinner: Mock Taco Meat (see page 131)

Note: Mock Taco Meat can be added to a corn tortilla with greens, tomatoes, onions, and guacamole or just added to a bed of greens.

Daily Fact

Blenders and juicers are invaluable assets in the raw foodist's arsenal, but oftentimes carry a hefty price tag. Many whether it is better to purchase a blender first, or a juicer. There is no simple answer, but something to consider is your lifestyle. A juicer will remove as much nutritional content as possible, and is easiest for the body to digest. A blender's delicious smoothies can take a few hours for the body to digest fully. Both provide all the nutrition you need, so it really is a question of personal preference!

Daily Affirmation

"I wake up feeling clear and energized in the morning . . . What is most profound for me about this light eating pattern is the flow of cosmic energy I feel coursing through my body. . . . During the day it feels as if joy is simply running through every cell independent of external factors."

—GABRIEL COUSENS, M.D. (raw food medical doctor),
Conscious Eating (North Atlantic Books, Berkeley, CA, 2000)

Challenger Notes / Log Entries

_____

_____

_____

_____

DAY 14

Recipes

Breakfast: Cinnamon Morning Smoothie (see page 76)

Lunch: Spicy Tropical Jicama Salsa & Salad (see page 100)

Dinner: Trine's Seed Burgers (see page 133)

Daily Fact

Dehydrated food maintains all the important nutritional content of raw food, while delivering it in a satisfying, addictive crunchy format. So if you're finding that juices and smoothies are still leaving you feeling hungry, try keeping a supply of crisps and crackers around to curb cravings!

Daily Affirmation

"If your blood is formed from eating the foods I teach [fruits and green-leaf vegetables] . . . . your soul will shout for joy and triumph over all misery of life. For the first time you will feel a vibration of vitality through your body (like a slight electric current) that shakes you delightfully."

—ARNOLD EHRET, *Mucusless Diet Healing System* (Benedict Lust Public., NY, 1970)

. . . From Real Raw Challengers

"14 days, and 100% Raw, I have dropped 9 pounds! I feel energized, and my body feels amazing! [T]his challenge . . . showed me that I didn't need certain things, that I could live without them and that my body benefited so very much from the challenge. Do it yourself, and do it for yourself."

—TIFFANY EDWARDS

Challenger Notes / Log Entries

_____

_____

_____

DAY 15

Recipes
Breakfast: Melon Morning (see page 77)

Lunch: Asian Slaw (see page 116)

Dinner: Sun Burgers (see page 135)

Daily Fact
Banish indigestion by eating raw food. Raw foodists experience a marked improvement in digestion. Cooked foods can contain sticky fat compounds that are harder to break down in the gut.

Daily Affirmation
"To me it is deeply moving that the same food choices that give us the best chance to eliminate world hunger are also those that take the least toll on the environment, contribute the most to our long-term health, are the safest, and are also, far and away, the most compassionate towards our fellow creatures."

—JOHN ROBBINS, author of *Diet for a New America* and
The Food Revolution

. . . From Real Raw Challengers
"When I began my two week challenge, my goal was to increase my energy level, clear my skin, initiate better digestion, and maintain optimal health. This journey, as I knew with any habit change, would be difficult. [But] on the third and fourth day, I felt a greater sense of energy in the afternoons and my skin was starting to reflect a healthier glow."

—KRIS SCHAFFER

Challenger Notes / Log Entries

DAY 16

Recipes
Breakfast: Tomato Watermelon Juice (see page 78)

Lunch: Pad Thai Salad (see page 108)

Dinner: Cauliflower Sushi Rolls (see page 136)

Daily Fact
Think big by thinking small! Some of the most nutritious content a raw foodist can partake of comes in the smallest package—algae, particularly blue-green algae, provides nutrients that are hardly found anywhere else! In fact, one of the most nutritious raw foods on the planet is a blue-green algae harvested from Klamath Lake in Oregon. This primordial plant life contains nutrients that will synergize your mind and your nervous system, increasing health *and* mental acuity!

Daily Affirmation
"My name is Valya. Raw food has been my lifestyle since I was eight years old in 1994. Before I changed my diet, I had a serious case of asthma. Every other night it would keep me from sleeping. I was supposed to have this steadily worsening breathing disorder for the rest of my life. Since the day I changed my diet, I have never had an asthmatic attack again. I'm so grateful that I don't have to suffer with this illness anymore! I will always cherish the freedom of being healthy. "

— Testimonial from www.rawfamily.com/testimonials

Challenger Notes / Log Entries

DAY 17

Recipes
Breakfast: V3 (see page 79)

Lunch: Curried Carrot Pâté (see page 105)

Dinner: Basic Spring Mix Salad (see page 144) with your choice of dressing

Daily Fact
Sprouting is the practice of growing seeds by soaking, draining, then rinsing at regular intervals until they germinate or sprout. Although slightly labor intensive, sprouts are highly dense in nutrients and a great way to grow your own food at home.

Daily Affirmation
"Nothing's changed my life more. I feel better about myself as a person, being conscious and responsible for my actions and I lost weight and my skin cleared up and I got bright eyes and I just became stronger and healthier and happier. Can't think of anything better in the world to be but be vegan."

—ALICIA SILVERSTONE

Challenger Notes / Log Entries

_____

_____

_____

_____

_____

_____

_____

_____

_____

DAY 18

Recipes
Breakfast: Pomegranate Orange Juice (see page 80)

Lunch: Carrot-Pulp Crackers (see page 110) with your choice of pâté

Dinner: Sauerkraut (see page 148)

Daily Fact
If everyone in the world would stop eating meat, there would be enough grain available to feed the world population (at least) seven times! If every person in the world would stop eating meat just one day a week, they would save grains equivalent to feed our world population of 7 billion. Just imagine.

Daily Affirmation
"My refusing to eat meat occasioned inconveniency, and I have been frequently chided for my singularity. But my light repast allows for greater progress, for greater clearness of head and quicker comprehension."

—BENJAMIN FRANKLIN

. . . From Real Raw Challengers
"I tried to lose weight all my life and sometimes it seemed to be working, but I was never satisfied with the amount of weight I lost or how long it took. When I decided to go raw I never expected to achieve this weight loss so fast. I also never expected to feel this great physically. I still have energy and don't feel like I am dieting but learning a whole new way of life."

—JANET BUSHBY

Challenger Notes / Log Entries

_____

_____

_____

_____

DAY 19

Recipes
Breakfast: Creamsicle® Morning (see page 81)

Lunch: GOT Crackers (see page 99), stack crackers with tomato slices, sprouts, or greens, and pâté for a raw BLT

Dinner: Live Un-Stir-Fry with Cauliflower "Rice" (see page 137)

Daily Fact
Wheatgrass contains most of the vitamins and minerals needed for human health. It's a whole meal and complete protein, with about 30 enzymes. It has up to 70% chlorophyll (which builds the blood). It's an excellent source of calcium, iron, magnesium, phosphorus, potassium, and zinc. Wheatgrass cleanses the body (natural raw detoxer) and it eliminates body and breath odors. The natural value of wheatgrass juice is so high that many people don't feel the "cravings" that lead to overeating. It's great for the skin, too.

Daily Affirmation
"Tis in ourselves that we are thus or thus. Our bodies are our gardens, to the which our wills are gardeners."

—WILLIAM SHAKESPEARE, *Othello,* Act 1, Scene 3

Challenger Notes / Log Entries

_____

_____

_____

_____

_____

_____

DAY 20

Recipes
Breakfast: Apple Avocado Mousse (see page 65)

Lunch: Summer Squash Slaw (see page 159)

Dinner: Basic Kale Salad (see page 143)

Daily Fact

Tibetan goji berries are extremely rich in antioxidants which help protect the cells in our bodies from diseases like cancer. They're also an excellent source of vitamin C and soluble fiber. They have more amino acids than bee pollen, more beta-carotene than carrots, more iron than spinach, and 21 trace minerals.

Daily Affirmation

"Bad men live that they may eat and drink, whereas good men eat and drink that they may live."

—SOCRATES

. . . From Real Raw Challengers

Everything about the way I ate changed. I ate more vegetables, more fruit, was introduced to gluten free products, and started eating avocados as a snack. It was GREAT! I felt great, slept better, and my skin cleared up. I didn't have energy crashes in the middle of the day or after I ate lunch. I felt stronger in all areas of my life."

—DAVE SCULLY

Challenger Notes / Log Entries

_____

_____

_____

DAY 21

Recipes
Breakfast: Apple Pear Juice (see page 83)

Lunch: Pumpkin Seed Pâté (see page 104) with salad greens

Dinner: Raw Vegan Lasagna Vegetable Stacks (see page 139)

Daily Fact
Hemp is one of the purest, most complete plants on earth. It has the perfect balance of Omega 3 and 6 for sustainable human health. This makes raw hemp seeds incredibly powerful against cancer. It might be the single best food to prevent it. It's a high quality, complete raw food protein, and has a massive trace mineral content.

It's the only seed that doesn't need to be germinated before eating: it has no enzyme exhibitors. Therefore it's easy to absorb.

Daily Affirmation
"If you can organize your kitchen, you can organize your life."

—LOUIS PARRISH

Challenger Notes / Log Entries

_____

_____

_____

_____

_____

_____

_____

_____

_____

DAY 22

Recipes

Breakfast: Pumpkin Spice and Everything Nice Smoothie (see page 84)

Lunch: Creamy Cucumber Soup (see page 121)

Dinner: Raw Thai Curry (see page 141)

Daily Fact

Raw foods provide organic skin care. If you've been gradually increasing your raw food intake throughout your challenge, you're likely seeing a change for the better in your complexion.

Daily Affirmation

"If a man earnestly seeks a righteous life, his first act of abstinence is from animal food."

—LEO TOLSTOY

. . . From Real Raw Challengers

"I've been eating raw foods ever since I can remember. My six siblings and I would venture into the woods and pick huckleberries, raspberries, blueberries, and teaberries. Now after raising my four children, I utilize my patio deck and flower beds to grow herbs, tomatoes, and sweet peppers. I also shop at local orchards and farms to prepare my daily raw food meals."

—MARY SCHAFFER

Challenger Notes / Log Entries

_____

_____

_____

_____

_____

DAY 23

Recipes
Breakfast: Almond & Cashew Milk (see page 85)

Lunch: Almond Hummus (see page 110), on greens or in a wrap using collard leaves or a flax wrap

Dinner: Basic Kale Salad (see page 143)

Daily Fact
Eating raw almonds can lower cholesterol. In a study by the University of Toronto, it found that eating 73 grams of raw almonds a day significantly lowered LDL or bad cholesterol by up to 12%.

Daily Affirmation
"To eat is a necessity, but to eat intelligently is an art."

—LA ROCHEFOUCAULD

Challenger Notes / Log Entries

_____

_____

_____

_____

_____

_____

_____

_____

_____

_____

_____

DAY 24

Recipes
Breakfast: Cashew or Brazil Nut Milk (see page 86)

Lunch: Pumpkin Seed Pâté (see page 104) with greens

Dinner: Karen's Zucchini Chips with Pumpkin Seed Pâté (see page 104)

Daily Fact
Maca is a dish-like fruit that grows in Peru. It's one of the top five super foods enjoyed by raw foodists. It's extraordinarily rich in nutrients: 10% protein, 60% carbohydrate, and is full of fatty acids, vitamins, and minerals.

The Peruvian root works gradually, not instantly. You need to eat maca continually to receive the full benefits. For the best results look for organic, raw maca powder.

Daily Affirmation
"Let your food be your medicine, and your medicine be your food."

—HIPPOCRATES

... From Real Raw Challengers
"I woke up before the alarm clock and felt really good! I can't tell you how long it has been since I woke up feeling refreshed! An average day for me would be half asleep at my desk around 3 p.m., staring at the clock praying for 5 o'clock. Now, the circles under my eyes are fading and they don't seem as puffy! Maybe there is some truth to this good clean living!"

—TAMMY JEROME

Challenger Notes / Log Entries

_____

_____

_____

DAY 25

Recipes
Breakfast: Coconut Milk (see page 87)

Lunch: Truly Raw Coleslaw (see page 146) with greens

Dinner: Chili Con Amore (see page 145)

Daily Fact
Many celebrities swear by a raw food diet. Demi Moore, Woody Harrelson, Alicia Silverstone have all evangelised about the benefits of a raw food diet. In fact Woody Harrelson has his own website on alternative living, environmental issues, as well as lots of information about raw food.

Daily Affirmation
"Until man duplicates a blade of grass, nature can laugh at his so-called scientific knowledge. Remedies from chemicals will never stand in favour compared with the products of nature, the living cell of the plant, the final result of the rays of the sun, the mother of all life."

—Thomas Edison

Challenger Notes / Log Entries

DAY 26

Recipes
Breakfast: Green Apple Smoothie (see page 88)
Lunch: Very Green Soup (see page 112)
Dinner: Sprouted Kamut Sushi (see page 142)

Daily Fact
Tryptophan is an amino acid which produces serotonin. Raw foods are great for your moods. Foods containing tryptophan include walnuts, figs, papaya, banana, strawberries, sweet cherries, mango, pineapple, grapefruit, and hazelnuts.

Daily Affirmation
"People who lack the clarity, courage, or determination to follow their own dreams will often find ways to discourage yours. When you change for the better, the people around you will be inspired to change also . . . but only after doing their best to make you stop. Live your truth and don't EVER stop."

—STEVE MARABOLI, *Life, the Truth, and Being Free*

. . . From Real Raw Challengers
"I find that I am sleeping better and not snoring as much as I used to and my energy level has increased. I have been told by quite a few people that I am "glowing" and my skin looks great. This was a great experience and I would tell anyone who is interested to definitely try it even if raw does not become a lifestyle they pursue."

—PHYLLIS TERRY

Challenger Notes / Log Entries

DAY 27

Recipes

Breakfast: Fresh Fruit Salad with Macadamia Cream (see page 73)

Lunch: Mary's Mixed Green Salad (see page 113)

Dinner: Brazil Nut Pâté (see page 152) with greens, in a wrap, on a cracker, or stuffed in celery

Daily Fact

Marianne Thieme, member of the Dutch parliament since 1996 estimated in 2010 that eating a vegetarian diet will reduce the world's CO_2 emission by 58% (if more humans become vegetarian)!

Daily Affirmation

"Pain is temporary. It may last a minute, or an hour, or a day, or a year, but eventually it will subside and something else will take its place. If I quit, however, it lasts forever. That surrender, even the smallest act of giving up, stays with me. So when I feel like quitting, I ask myself, which would I rather live with?"

—LANCE ARMSTRONG

Challenger Notes / Log Entries

_____

_____

_____

_____

_____

_____

_____

_____

DAY 28

Recipes
Breakfast: Blueberry Grape Smoothie (see page 89)
Lunch: Robert's New Life Salad (see page 114)
Dinner: Spicy BBQ Zucchini Chips (see page 157)

Daily Fact
Raw food hygiene is very important. Cooking destroys many of the bacteria such as E. coli, which are potentially harmful to humans. So be extra careful and vigilant when eating strictly raw.

Daily Affirmation
"Every man who has ever been earnest to preserve his higher or poetic faculties in the best condition has been particularly inclined to abstain from animal food."

—HENRY DAVID THOREAU

. . . From Real Raw Challengers
"Determined to keep my family truly healthy, I submerged myself in raw cookbooks and joined a raw potluck and support group hosted by Living Dynamically's Lisa Montgomery. Eventually, navigating through the organics aisle became easier, green juice became palatable, and most importantly—[my husband's arthritis] was feeling better."

—LINDA COOPER

Challenger Notes / Log Entries

_____

_____

_____

_____

DAY 29

Recipes

Breakfast: Strawberry Coconut Milk (see page 90)

Lunch: Apple and Butternut Squash Raw Soup (see page 122)

Dinner: Basic Spring Mix Salad (see page 144) with pumpkin seed oil dressing

Daily Fact

Squash provides notable amounts of energy giving complex carbohydrates, as well as omega-3 fatty acids, folate, niacin, copper, tryptophan, manganese, and dietary fiber. Moreover, apples can provide important benefits for nearly every system in the human body, including neurological (through the prevention of dementia), cardiovascular (by decreasing blood cholesterol levels), digestive (by supporting colon and intestinal health and regulating metabolism), as well as reproductive (through the prevention of prostate cancer).

Daily Affirmation

"Nature itself is the best physician."

—HIPPOCRATES

Challenger Notes / Log Entries

DAY 30

Recipes

Breakfast: Pineapple Smoothie (see page 91)

Lunch: Mellow Kim Chi (see page 115)

Dinner: Creamy Lemon, Dill & Garlic Salad Dressing/Dip (see page 167), can be used with crudités or on greens

Daily Fact

Having completed thirty days of a raw food diet, you've laid the perfect foundation for expanding into other areas of healthy living! Even if exercise regimens have failed you in the past, a raw food diet should leave you feeling brighter, lighter, and more energetic! You already managed something amazing in completing this 30-day challenge, who knows what else you can accomplish? Congratulations, and good luck!

Daily Affirmation

"Great spirits have always found violent opposition from mediocrities. The latter cannot understand it when a man does not thoughtlessly submit to hereditary prejudices, but honestly and courageously uses his intelligence and fulfills the duty to express the results of his thought in clear form."

—ALBERT EINSTEIN

. . . From Real Raw Challengers

"...It was not an overnight transformation. I feel a sense of compassion and patience is valuable throughout the process. My advice to seekers is to start small, start right now, and be bold in asking for help! Health foodies love to talk about food! Blessings on your journey."

—SALLY BOWDLE

Challenger Notes / Log Entries

PART III:
RAW RECIPES

Almond Milk Smoothie

(Kimberton Whole Foods, www.kimbertonwholefoods.com)

Soak: Almonds, 8 hours or overnight
Prep: Almond milk, 10–15 minutes
 Smoothie, 7 minutes

Almond Milk

2 cups, raw almonds,
 strained

2–3 cups spring water

Vanilla, non-alcoholic;
 I use 2 teaspoons or
 more as I love vanilla

12 Medjool dates, pitted

6 cups water, pure

Smoothie

1 tray ice cubes

3 bananas, peeled

4–6 ounces blueberries

Almond milk, enough to
 cover all of the above in
 your blender

1 tablespoon raw honey

Raw cacao powder, to taste

Almond Milk

Let almonds soak overnight in water (for better digestion). In the morning rinse and drain the almonds. Then put them in your blender or jar. Add 2–3 cups of clean (spring) water along with the vanilla, dates, and a pinch of salt. Blend well. Pour the almond milk in the nut bag or through cheesecloth. It's easiest if you have a large bowl underneath to catch the filtered milk. Now holding the bag with one hand, squeeze out the additional milk with your other hand.

Tip: If you dehydrate the almond pulp, you can use it to make raw cakes and cookies. Many save it in the fridge for about 2 days (shake before drinking), although I prefer to drink it fresh. You can buy nut bags at most health stores and online. You can also use nylons, cheesecloth, or a paint strainer.

Smoothie

Place all of the smoothie ingredients in a Vitamix® blender, pouring in the almond milk last. (I pour in enough to cover all of the ingredients and depending on how thirsty I am I may keep adding a bit more.) Blend all of the ingredients until desired consistency is reached. If you like your smoothie to have texture, then don't blend it very long. If you want your blend to be very smooth then blend the mixture a bit longer.

The wonderful thing about smoothies is that you can make a batch for the day and store them in ball jars and drink them the rest of the day.

Also you can add all sorts of goodies to your smoothies like maca, goji berries, nutritional powders, protein powders... basically you can get carried away with what you add.

Apple Avocado Mousse

(Kimberton Whole Foods, www.kimbertonwholefoods.com)

Prep: 15 minutes
Serves 2

1 avocado
2 apples, peeled and cored
¼ cup purified water

Take the avocado meat out of the avocado. Combine the apple and avocado in a mixing bowl. Mix apple, avocado, and water with a hand mixer. Drizzle in the water as you go, just in case you don't need all of it.

Young Thai Coconut Smoothie
(Lisa Montgomery)

Prep: 7 minutes

1 young Thai Coconut, meat and liquid
1 tray of ice cubes (optional)
3 bananas
4–6 ounces fresh fruit
1 tablespoon raw honey
Handful of cacao nibs

Blend all of the above ingredients in a Vitamix® high-speed blender.

Note: Some people don't like ice in their smoothies because it makes it too cold. If you don't like ice, you can simply leave it out of the recipe. You can also freeze your fruit before using.

> *I had taken many years of classes before I could figure out how to open a young Thai coconut that would work for me. Because of my lengthy challenge I wanted to show the Challengers how easy it really is to open the coconut . . . or at least the easy method I now use. I take the heel of a cheap cleaver that I bought at my local Asian market and just make a circle cutting around the top of the coconut, pop the lid off and pour the liquid into the Vitamix® blender. I use an ice cream scoop to get the meat out of the coconut. I can now open a coconut within minutes where in the past it would take me so long that I would give up.*

Water-Based Smoothie

(Lisa Montgomery)

For those of you who may not want to make almond milk or who do not want to learn how to open a young Thai coconut, this water-based smoothie is a perfect alternative.

Prep: 5 minutes

4–6 ounces fresh or frozen strawberries, with stems
2 oranges, peeled, quartered
Handful of greens
3 bananas
1 tray of ice cubes
Water, to cover ingredients
1 tablespoon raw honey

Place all of the ingredients in a Vitamix® blender and cover with clean, fresh spring water and blend.

Thanks to Victoria Boutenko, everyone loves green smoothies. Feel free to throw greens into any of the smoothies you make to get additional greens in your diet.

Tammy's Breakfast Smoothie

(Tammy Jerome)

Prep: 5 minutes

6 large strawberries
2 medium bananas
1 handful of red grapes
1 handful of blueberries
1 8-ounce glass ice cubes
½ to 1 cup water (depending on desired consistency—less
    water for a thicker smoothie or more water for a thinner
    smoothie)

Combine ingredients in a Vitamix® high-speed blender until blended.

Note: This recipe makes enough smoothies for about 2 glasses. I sometimes also put it into small plastic containers and freeze them for a healthy ice cream snack. Yummy!

Karen's Morning Snacks

(Dr. Karen Izzi)

Soak: Seeds, 4 hours
Prep: 15 minutes

4 medium dried apricots, diced
1 cup raw cashews
1 medium pear, chopped up in bite size pieces
1 medium carrot, chopped up in bite size pieces
¼ cup water
¾ cup raw, soaked pumpkin seeds
¾ cup raw, soaked sunflower seeds
1 teaspoon cinnamon
1 tablespoon chia seeds
¼ cup flaxseeds
½ raw oats
½ shredded coconut

Combine all ingredients in a Vitamix® high-speed blender or a food processor until blended to desired consistency. Form into bars.

This is a great snack for when you're on the go, as well as for breakfast.

My preferred consistency is to pulse the combined the ingredients so it's more a munchy crunchy, hand-to-mouth consistency but some may want it totally blended so it's more of a drink. Try it both ways (or somewhere in between) and see what works for you. The taste is great no matter what consistency you prefer.

Granny Granola

(Dr. Karen Izzi)

Prep: 15 minutes
Dehydrate: 10 hours at 105°F

3 Granny Smith apples, diced
1 cup raw oats
1 cup almonds, slivered
1 cup pumpkin seeds
1 cup sunflower seeds
1 cup raisins
2 tablespoons honey
1 tablespoon agave nectar
½ teaspoon cinnamon
½ cup water, if needed

Toss all ingredients in a large bowl, coating fruit and nuts. Dehydrate for about 10 hours.

Nuts About Granola
(Sheryll Chavarria, Raw Can Roll Cafe)

Soak: 24 hours
Prep: 20 minutes
Dehydrate: 24 hours at 115°F

3 cups walnuts or pecans
8 cups steel cut oats (soaked overnight)
    or buckwheat groats (soaked for 4 hours)
5 cup banana purée
2½ cups agave
¼ cup vanilla extract
Pinch Celtic sea salt

Put nuts into food processor until coarsely processed. Mix all ingredients together and spread mixture out onto Teflex sheets on top of Dehydrator trays. Dehydrate for 24 hours or more at 115°F.

    Serve with a nut milk and fresh-cut fruit. You can also try topping it with blueberries, which make a nice color contrast.

Raw Banana Pancakes

(Kimberton Whole Foods, www.kimbertonwholefoods.com)

Soak: 4 hours
Prep: 20 minutes
Dehydrate (optional): 105°F, as desired

2 cups pine nuts,
2 cups pecans, soaked
2 whole bananas, ripe
1 cup water
½ cup Medjool dates, soaked
1-inch vanilla bean, chopped
½ pinch sea salt (optional)

In a high-speed blender, combine all ingredients. Blend well until the batter is thoroughly mixed. Serve with raw maple syrup, honey, or fruit (if desired). The batter will keep in the refrigerator for several days.

Optional: Dehydrate at 105°F for warmth and for greater pancake effect.

Fresh Fruit Salad with Macadamia Cream

(Kimberton Whole Foods, www.kimbertonwholefoods.com)

Prep: 15 minutes

Chopped fruit of your choice
One handful of raw macadamia nuts
Juice of half an orange (or a whole one juiciness)
2–4 large Medjool dates (or 4–8 smaller soaked ones)
Small piece of vanilla bean (optional)

Prepare your fruit salad using a wide range of fresh, juicy fruits of your choice. (A good mixture might be banana, orange, apple, strawberries, nectarines, and blueberries.) Next, make your topping by blending remaining ingredients together until a thick creamy mixture is created. Taste before using and adjust ingredients according to your preference. You may want to add a pinch of salt just to bring out the flavors a little more.

Serve the fruit salad topped with a good dose of the macadamia cream. The topping recipe will keep for about 2–3 days in the refrigerator.

Great for topping some breakfasts for something a bit more sustaining. Or why not throw a tablespoon or two of it into your fruit smoothie?

Lisa's Every Day Green Drink

(Lisa Montgomery)

Prep: 7 minutes

½ lemon, cut to fit into juicer
1 cucumber, cut into spears to fit into juicer
4 celery stalks
Handful of greens
6 apples, cut to fit into juicer

Feed all ingredients into a Tribest Green Star Elite juicer.

Note: You can adjust the above ingredients or even toss in some additional vegetables such as carrots, ginger, cabbage, or beets.

Vanilla Crème Smoothie

(Lisa Montgomery)

Prep: 5 minutes

3 peeled bananas
1 tablespoon Singing Dog® vanilla, alcohol free
9 dates, pitted
1 tablespoon raw honey
16 ounces almond milk
1 tray ice

Combine ingredients in a Vitamix® high-speed blender until desired consistency is reached.

> *I always add aloe vera juice and liquid trace minerals to my breakfast smoothies.*
>
> *If a tray of ice is too chilling for you, then freeze your bananas for cooling and add water to equal the amount of one tray of ice.*

Cinnamon Morning Smoothie
(Lisa Montgomery)

Prep: 5 minutes

4 ounces frozen organic raspberries
½–1 tablespoon Red Ape Cinnamon™
8 ounces almond milk
3 bananas
1 tablespoon raw honey
1 tray ice cubes

Combine ingredients in a Vitamix® high-speed blender until desired consistency is reached.

Melon Morning

(Lisa Montgomery)

Prep: 5 minutes

3 cups watermelon fruit
1 piece watermelon rind

Run the watermelon fruit and rind through a Tribest Fruitstar juicer or Tribest Green Star juicer.

Tomato Watermelon Juice

(Lisa Montgomery)

Prep: 5 minutes

2 cups watermelon fruit
2 medium to large tomatoes

Chop up the ingredients and run it through a Tribest Fruitstar juicer and serve.

The tomato in this recipe adds a little salty spice to the watermelon's sweetness so that they balance each other out.

V3

(Lisa Montgomery)

Prep: 5 minutes

3 medium to large tomatoes
¾ cup green pepper
1 stalk celery
Sea salt, to taste

Run ingredients through a Tribest Fruitstar juicer, stir, and drink.

    Note: If you want to spice it up you could add a pinch of cayenne or Tabasco sauce (which is not raw or fresh).

Pomegranate Orange Juice

(Lisa Montgomery)

Prep: 5 minutes

4 oranges, peeled
½ cup fresh pomegranate seeds

Run oranges and pomegranate seeds through a Tribest Fruitstar juicer. Stir and drink.

Pomegranates are great for you, but they tend to be a little bitter. When you combine them with the sweetness of the oranges, it's a perfect match made in fruit heaven.

This drink is cool and refreshing. I love it!

Creamsicle® Morning

(Lisa Montgomery)

I used to love eating Creamsicles® growing up, so this is how I get my fix.

Prep: 5 minutes

1–2 oranges, peeled
1–2 cups almond milk
3 bananas
1 tablespoon Singing Dog® vanilla
1 tray ice cubes

Combine ingredients in a Vitamix® high-speed blender and serve.

Neapolitan Smoothie

(Lisa Montgomery)

Prep: 5 minutes

8 ounces strawberries, with stems

1–2 tablespoons raw cacao

1–2 tablespoons Singing Dog® vanilla or Sun Organic™ vanilla

12 ounces almond milk

3 bananas

1 tray ice cubes

1 tablespoon raw honey

Combine ingredients in a Vitamix® high-speed blender.

Apple Pear Juice
(Lisa Montgomery)

Prep: 5 minutes

3 apples, size cut to fit through juicer
3 pears, size cut to fit through juicer

Run apples and pears through a Tribest Green Star Elite juicer, stir, and drink.

This drink is clean and refreshing. It's also super easy to make! There's no need to core or remove the stems on the fruit, you can run them right through the juicer and have homemade juice in seconds.

Pumpkin Spice and Everything Nice Smoothie

(Lisa Montgomery)

Prep: 5 minutes

3 bananas

4 ounces fruit, pumpkin, or butternut squash

1 tablespoon raw honey

1 tray ice cubes

8 to 12 ounces almond milk

½ to 1 teaspoon pumpkin spice, or to taste

Combine the ingredients in aVitamix® high-speed blender and blend until desired consistency is reached.

Pumpkin spice typically includes cinnamon, ginger, clove, and nutmeg. If you don't have pumpkin spice at home, but have the individual spices on hand you can come up with your own blend.

Almond & Cashew Milk

(Lisa Montgomery)

Soak: Raw almonds, 8 hours or overnight
Prep: 5 minutes

1 cup raw soaked raw almonds
1 cup raw cashews
1 tablespoon alcohol-free vanilla
12 Medjool dates, pitted
6 cups water

Combine ingredients in Vitamix® high-speed blender until thoroughly blended. Place nut bag over a large bowl. Pour mixture through nut bag and milk the bag. The liquid that comes out through the nut bag will now become your milk. Store milk in the refrigerator in a ½ gallon canning jar with lid. You can also save the pulp and turn it into crackers, croutons, or scones.

Cashew or Brazil Nut Milk

(Lisa Montgomery)

Prep: 5 minutes

2 cups raw cashews or 2 cups Brazil nuts
1 tablespoon alcohol-free vanilla
12 Medjool dates, pitted
6 cups water

Combine ingredients in Vitamix® high-speed blender until thoroughly blended. Place nut bag over a large bowl. Pour mixture through nut bag and milk the bag. The liquid that comes out through the nut bag will now become your milk. Store milk in the refrigerator in a ½ gallon canning jar with lid. You can also save the pulp and turn it into crackers, croutons, or scones.

Coconut Milk and Coconut Water

(Lisa Montgomery)

Prep: 5 minutes

1 young Thai coconut

Use the back end of a cleaver knife and cut a circle around the top of the coconut.

To make coconut water, simply pour the liquid from the young Thai coconut.

For coconut milk, blend the coconut water and the meat (which you can remove from the inside of the coconut using an ice cream scoop) and combine them together in a Vitamix® high-speed blender.

Green Apple Smoothie
(Lisa Montgomery)

Prep: 5 minutes

2 green apples, quartered and cored
Handful of greens
3 bananas
1 tablespoon raw honey
1 tray of ice cubes
16 ounces water

Combine ingredients in a Vitamix® high-speed blender until smooth. Blend and drink.

Blueberry Grape Smoothie

(Lisa Montgomery)

Prep: 5 minutes

½ cup frozen or fresh grapes
½ cup frozen or fresh blueberries
3 bananas, peeled
1 young Thai coconut (meat and juice)
1 tray ice cubes
1 tablespoon raw honey

Combine ingredients together in a Vitamix® high-speed blender until smooth. (If you don't have a high-speed blender, you can use whatever blender you have on hand.)

Strawberry Coconut Milk
(Lisa Montgomery)

Prep: 5 minutes

6 ounces strawberries, fresh or frozen
1 young Thai coconut (meat and liquid)
1 tablespoon vanilla
1 tablespoon raw honey
3 bananas
1 tray ice cubes

Combine ingredients together in a Vitamix® high-speed blender until smooth.

Pineapple Smoothie

(Lisa Montgomery)

Prep: 5 minutes

1 1½-inch thick slice of fresh pineapple
3 bananas
1 tablespoon raw honey
1 tray of ice cubes
12 ounces almond milk

Blend ingredients together in a Vitamix® high-speed blender until smooth.

Tammy's Fruit Salad
(Tammy Jerome)

Prep: 30 minutes

1 personal size seedless watermelon
1 cantaloupe
1 honeydew melon
1 pound red grapes
1 (16 ounce) container strawberries, sliced in quarters
1 (16 ounce) container blueberries
3 kiwis (fruit), to be used as garnish

Use a melon baller to cut the watermelon and cantaloupe. Combine all ingredients. Be sure to wash all fruit before handling and adding to your salad!

Sprout Salad

(Chef Barbara Shevkun,
Rawfully Tempting)

Prep: 15 minutes
Sprouting: Mung beans and
lentils, 3 days

2 cups sprouted mung beans
    (¼ cup mung beans before
    sprouted)
1 cup sprouted lentils (¼ cup
    lentils before sprouting)
1 apple, sliced
½ to 1 cup finely chopped
    golden beets, peeled
½ cup raisins
2 tablespoons sauerkraut (such as Bubbies®)

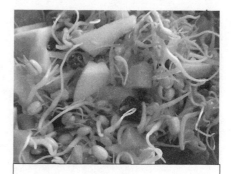

Photo courtesy of Chef Barbara
Shevkun, Rawfully Tempting
(www.rawfullytempting.com)

Combine all ingredients. You can also add avocado, greens, mangoes, or any of your favorite vegetables. Top with your favorite
dressing. (I added a spoonful of juice from the Bubbies® sauerkraut
and it was delicious!)

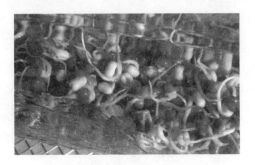

*Photo courtesy of Chef Barbara
Shevkun, Rawfully Tempting
(www.rawfullytempting.com)*

SPROUTING: LENTILS, GARBANZOS, AND MUNG BEANS, OH MY!

(Chef Barbara Shevkun, Rawfully Tempting)

Beans, beans, beans. We've got lentils, garbanzo beans, and mung beans and it's time to do some sprouting. There are many health benefits to eating sprouts and I've read that sprouting increases enzymes up to 600%. I don't know if that's true, but I do know they feel good and my body tells me what's good and what's not. It says, "Sprouts are *good*!"

SPROUTING:

Rinse beans really well in a strainer and place them in a large jar. Fill with filtered water (you can also do this in a strainer and cover with a towel).

Close jar and let sit overnight, or all day (8–12 hours). Preferably, rinse and change water once during that time.

Drain sprouts, rinse, and drain again. Use sprouting lids (using screens, cheesecloth, or paper towels and a rubber band) to cover jars and set aside, away from direct light. Lay jars down, preferably tilted to drain any excess water (a dish drain works great for this).

Many experts suggest rinsing and draining every 8 to 12 hours, but I prefer to rinse every few hours. Sprouts can be ready in 2 to 4 days (I usually like the tails to not be any longer than the bean itself, but this can vary). For chickpeas, bite into one. If it's tender and easy to bite into, it's done and there may only be a bud of a tail. Mung beans sprout very quickly, so if they taste good, they are done.

When your beans are done sprouting, do a final rinse and drain *really* well before placing them in an airtight container in the refrigerator.

Other uses: Chickpeas are great in raw vegan hummus, and I also like to mix mine with cashews. Believe it or not, chickpeas are also great when blended into cookie or brownie mixes because they add a wonderfully chewy, cake-like texture. My favorite sprouts in salad are mung beans, lentils, and broccoli.

Horseradish & Dill Crackers/Bread

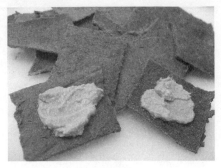

(Chef Barbara Shevkun, Rawfully Tempting)
As part of my recent exploration into my "roots," I prepared fresh horseradish. It was deeply earthy and delicious. From that recipe, I made a horseradish hummus dip, which was lighter in texture, but also fabulous. I needed some crunchy crackers, so what else? Horseradish & Dill Crackers, of course! The horseradish flavor turned out rather mild while the dill seems to permeate the crackers. I love dill, so it works for me, and I can spread either horseradish or the hummus on them. If you're not a fan of dill, replace it with your favorite herb. This recipe may also be prepared as a bread.

Photo courtesy of Chef Barbara Shevkun, Rawfully Tempting (www.rawfullytempting.com)

Soak: Walnuts, overnight
Prep: 20–30 minutes
Dehydrate: Approximately 24 hours or as desired, at 115°F

1½ cups walnuts (soaked overnight)
½ cup almond pulp/flour
1½ cups veggie pulp (from juicing), or zucchini, chopped
2½ cups water, or as needed
¼ cup ground flaxseed
3 tablespoons hemp seed

2 tablespoons grated horseradish (optional)
1 garlic clove, minced
1 teaspoon dill, dried (save ½ teaspoon for garnish) or 1½ tablespoons fresh dill
2 tablespoons sesame seeds (may also use some for garnish)

1 tablespoon lemon juice
1 tablespoon honey
(or your favorite
sweetener)
1 tablespoon Annie's
horseradish mustard
(optional, not raw)

¼ teaspoon onion powder
¼ teaspoon garlic powder
¾ teaspoon sea salt

In food processor, process walnuts, almond pulp, and veggie pulp.

Add water as needed to mix (if you use more water, the dehydration time will need to be increased). Add remaining ingredients and continue to process until well mixed. Taste and adjust seasoning to your liking. Spread 1 cup of batter onto no-stick dehydrator sheet, rotating the tray in a circle as you spread the batter onto the tray (an offset spatula helps a lot). Repeat this for each tray. Garnish with dill and/or sesame seeds, or poppy seeds, onion flakes, etc. Dehydrate at 115°F for about 3 hours. To flip over, place a mesh tray on top. Holding two trays together, quickly flip over. Remove tray and peel off non-stick sheet. Score batter using a dull-edged knife and continue to dehydrate 12–18 hours, or until crisp.

Note: For bread, spread batter onto two trays, instead of three, making the layers thicker than crackers. Follow directions above, although you may have to wait another hour to flip. Score into squares. Dehydrate until bread is firm, but not crunchy. Freeze in airtight container and use as needed.

Creamy Beet and Horseradish Dip
(Chef Barbara Shevkun, Rawfully Tempting)

Prep: 20 minutes

Horseradish
1½ cups horseradish root, chopped
½ medium red beet, chopped
½–¾ cup water (or more as needed)
2 tablespoons vinegar (or coconut water vinegar)
3 tablespoons maple syrup (grade B or your favorite sweetener)
⅛ teaspoon sea salt

Dip
3 tablespoons horseradish (see above)
¼ cup cashews, soaked 1–2 hours
¼ cup water (or as needed for consistency)
2 tablespoons Irish moss paste (optional)

Horseradish
Clean, peel, and chop horseradish root.

Add horseradish, beet, and water to blender or food processor to blend.

Add vinegar, maple syrup, and salt. Process until well blended.

Transfer to a glass jar or airtight container.

Dip
Blend cashews and water.

Add Irish moss paste, if available (optional, but it gives a little more body).

Transfer to a bowl and stir in horseradish (the more you use, the hotter the mix will be).

Serve with sliced cucumbers or other veggies, on raw vegan crackers, over salad, or use as a condiment in wraps. Delicious!

GOT (Garlic Onion Tomato) Crackers

(Denise DiJoseph)

These are great for introducing raw foods to newbies because the square shape is visually appealing and eases their mind and taste buds into accepting healthier substitutes.

Soak: Seeds, 8 hours
Prep: 30 minutes
Dehydrate: Approximately 24 hours or as desired at 105–110°F

1 cup ground flaxseed
1 cup sunflower seeds (presoaked 8 hours and drained)
3 medium to large yellow onions
¼ cup extra-virgin olive oil (such as Bariani®)
¼ cup frontier organic powdered tomato
4 garlic cloves minced in a garlic press (or to taste)
5 sundried tomatoes chopped (presoaked in water to soften)
3 tablespoons Bragg® Liquid Aminos (amino acids)

Combine all ingredients in a food processor. Scoop mixture onto Teflex sheets and smooth evenly with a spatula to create a giant square cracker. Dehydrate at 105–110°F. Check on it and turn it over, when possible, without breaking it. You can now add any optional seasoning if desired (see below). When the mushy mixture has dried and cracker has flexibility, you can let it continue drying or snip it into squares with kitchen shears, then return the crackers to the dehydrator until done to your preference.

Makes about 4–5 large squares. Break up the crackers into smaller bits if you chose not to snip them. Store in individual snack bags for portion control. Large batches can be vacuum sealed and stored in the freezer.

*Optional: To make a variety of flavors for an assorted cracker medley, sprinkle one tray of cracker mixture with a slight dusting of cayenne, another with basil, and another with oregano or any other seasonings you prefer. Leave at least one of the tray crackers plain.

Spicy Tropical Jicama Salsa & Salad

(Kimberton Whole Foods, www.kimbertonwholefoods.com)

Prep: 30 minutes

Salad
½ large pineapple, cut into small cubes
½ jicama, cut into small cubes
1 bunch cilantro, finely chopped
½ red onion, diced

Dressing
1 cup coconut milk (combine ⅔ cup coconut meat and 1 cup coconut water)

½ cup lime juice
4 tablespoons coconut nectar (or honey, maple syrup, agave)
½ teaspoon Himalayan pink salt
4–5 tablespoons coconut oil, warmed to liquid
½–1 teaspoon paprika
½–1 jalapeño (see note below)

Place all salad ingredients in a bowl and mix thoroughly. Place all dressing ingredients in a Vitamix® high-speed blender and blend until smooth. Pour dressing over salad and mix.

Salad will last 1–2 days in the refrigerator when dressed or 3–4 if dressing and salad are stored separately.

If you have a Vitamix® high-speed blender, you don't need to chop the jalapeño because the blender is powerful enough to chop up the pepper. If you are using a regular blender, you should chop the jalapeño before adding it to the blender, just in case it is not strong enough to blend the ingredients appropriately.

Popeye Would Be Jealous Crackers
(Dr. Karen Izzi)

Soak: Sunflower seeds, overnight or for 8 hours, and sprout for 3 days
Prep: 20–30 minutes
Dehydrate: At 105°F for 24 hours or until desired consistency is reached

16 ounces fresh spinach
1 cup onion, chopped
1 green bell pepper, chopped
1 teaspoon garlic powder
2 tablespoons nutritional yeast
1 cup ground flaxseeds
1 cup raw, sprouted sunflower seeds
Sea salt, to taste

Blend the spinach, onion, pepper, garlic powder, and nutritional yeast in processor until spinach is coarsely chopped. In a large bowl, stir in flaxseeds to create a thick paste. Add sunflower seeds and stir until blended. Smooth onto dehydrator mat, about ½ inch thick. Add sea salt to taste. Dehydrate at 105°F until crisp. Break into bite-size pieces. Enjoy. Store in a cool, dry place (unless they disappear first).

Sunflower Pâté

(Dr. Karen Izzi)

Soak: 8 hours
Prep: 20 minutes

2 cups raw, soaked sunflower seeds

5 large carrots

1 cup lemon juice

½ cup Bragg® Liquid Aminos (amino acids)

½ cup soy sauce or wheat free tamari

½ cup chopped scallions

2–4 slices red onion

4 tablespoons chopped parsley

¼ teaspoon ginger

¼ teaspoon cumin

½ teaspoon salt

Cayenne pepper, to taste

Combine ingredients in food processor with S blade until desired consistency is reached. This pâté can be served with greens, on a raw cracker such as Popeye's crackers, or as a dip.

Italian Eggplant Chips
(Dr. Karen Izzi)

Prep: 15 minutes
Dehydrate: Until crispy, at 105°F

2 tablespoons Bragg® Liquid Aminos (amino acids)
1 tablespoon olive oil
1 teaspoon oregano
½ teaspoon rosemary
½ teaspoon basil
1 teaspoon garlic, minced or pressed
½ teaspoon Celtic sea salt
1 small eggplant, sliced thin
3 tablespoons sesame seeds

In a small bowl, mix amino acids, olive oil, the fresh herbs, garlic, and sea salt. Coat each slice of eggplant with the mixture and lay on a dehydrator sheet. (I leave the skin on the eggplant so it becomes extra crunchy, but you can remove it if you prefer.)

Sprinkle sesame seeds on each slice. Dehydrate at 105°F until crispy.

Karen's Zucchini Chips

(Dr. Karen Izzi)

You can serve these with Karen's Sunflower Pâté and eat it as a lunch or dinner, or eat it plain as a crunchy snack.

Prep: 15 minutes
Dehydrate: Until crispy, at 105°F

1 tablespoon fresh dill, chopped
1 tablespoon garlic salt
1 tablespoon onion powder
1 tablespoon nutritional yeast

2 small zucchini, sliced thinly
2 tablespoons cold-pressed olive oil

Combine spices in a bowl. Dip zucchini slices in olive oil, roll in the spices, and place on Teflex-lined dehydrator tray. Dehydrate at 105°F until desired consistency is reached.

Pumpkin Seed Pâté

(Dr. Karen Izzi)

I love pâtés with greens as they add substance and fill you up. Plus they taste great as a dip, as a filler in celery sticks, or as a spoonful on a tomato slice or cucumber slice; they make great little appetizers.

Soak: Seeds, 4 hours
Prep: 20 minutes

1½ cups pumpkin seeds, soaked
1 bunch fresh chives
1 clove fresh garlic
1 teaspoon chili powder

1 teaspoon agave syrup
2 tablespoons tomato paste
2 tablespoons olive oil
½ teaspoon sea salt

Combine ingredients in a food processor using the S blade until desired consistency is reached.

Curried Carrot Pâté

(Kimberton Whole Foods, www.kimbertonwholefoods.com)

Prep: 15 minutes

2 organic carrots, grated and chopped
1 tablespoon raw organic peanut butter
1 teaspoon curry powder

Place all ingredients in a food processor and blend until pâté is formed. Pair with raw veggies for dipping or use as topping for other dishes. This pâté can also be placed with veggies on greens for lunch or in a wrap with veggies for a meal.

Root Salad

(Dr. Karen Izzi)

This recipe has been a hit ever since I created it, even at family parties. I served it to all of the people who think the way I eat is "weird" and they loved it! The longer it marinates the better it tastes.

Prep: 25 minutes

3 large carrots

1 medium daikon

6 medium white beets, cooked and cut into small sticks

1 cup fresh cilantro, finely chopped

1 tablespoon sesame oil

½ teaspoon garlic salt

2 tablespoons rice vinegar

Shred all ingredients in a food processor. Combine shredded ingredients in a bowl, toss, and serve.

Chilled Cucumber Mint Soup

(Ken Alan)

Prep: 15 minutes

2 large cucumbers, peeled and seeded
2 cups water
¼ cup raw sugar or raw honey
1 tablespoon salt
Dash of white pepper
½ cup sour cream
¼ cup fresh mint leaves
½ cup extra-virgin olive oil

Combine the cucumber and water in a blender. Purée mixture until smooth. Add sugar, salt, white pepper, sour cream, and fresh mint leaves. Continue to purée until all ingredients are completely incorporated. While blender is still on, slowly add the olive oil. Strain through a fine strainer. Store in refrigerator for at least 1 hour before serving. Serve with diced cucumber, mint sprig, and olive oil.

Note: For those of you who don't do dairy, you could substitute the sour cream with cashew, young Thai coconut meat, or avocado.

Pad Thai Salad
(Kimberton Whole Foods, www.kimbertonwholefoods.com)

Soak: Nuts, 8 hours
Prep: 25 minutes

2 zucchinis, sliced into strips with a vegetable peeler

2 large handfuls of bean sprouts, approximately 2 cups

¾ cup soaked nuts, chopped (use almonds, peanuts, or cashews)

1 red or yellow bell pepper, sliced into strips

4 green onions, diced

½ cup fresh chopped cilantro

Juice from one lime

1 tablespoon raw, cold-pressed olive oil

¼ teaspoon sea salt

Toss all ingredients together in a bowl until well coated. Add a dash more salt if desired and enjoy!

Happy Harvest Salad

(Lisa Montgomery)

I called this the "Happy Harvest Salad" because the harvest season is a perfect time to use the fresh ingredients from your own garden or your local farm stand.

Prep: 20 minutes

4 large tomatoes, chopped
¼ cup red onion, diced
3 cloves garlic, chopped
3 ears fresh corn, removed from cob
¼ cup basil, chiffonade
1 tablespoon Austria's Finest Naturally® Pumpkin Seed Oil
1 teaspoon Himalayan sea salt
Pinch cracked black pepper

Combine the above ingredients in a bowl, toss, and enjoy. I think this salad actually tastes better the next day. On the first day, the basil can sometimes taste overpowering but when the flavors have an opportunity to meld overnight, the flavors are balanced and really delicious.

Carrot-Pulp Crackers
(Mary Schaffer)

Soak: Seeds and groats, 6–8 hours
Prep: 25 minutes
Dehydrate: Approximately 24 hours at 105°F

⅓ cup buckwheat groats, soaked in water about 6–8 hours

1 tablespoon flaxseeds, soaked in water about 6–8 hours

1 cup carrot pulp from organic carrots

1½ tablespoons onion, minced

1 tablespoon garlic, minced

1 tablespoon hemp seeds

½ teaspoon salt (Celtic or Himalayan)

¼ cup organic cold-pressed olive oil

Mix all ingredients together in a medium-size bowl, then shape into squares. Put in the dehydrator at 105°F for 24 hours.

You can make a lunch out of these crackers by placing a pâté, greens, sprouts, and slices of tomatoes and onions in between crackers.

Almond Hummus
(Kimberton Whole Foods, www.kimbertonwholefoods.com)

Soak: Almonds, 8 hours
Prep: 15 minutes

2 cups almonds, soaked
½ cup tahini
1 large garlic clove, minced
Juice of 2 large lemons

¼ to ½ teaspoon sea salt
1 tablespoon fresh chopped parsley
1 teaspoon basil

Break down the almonds using a homogenizing juicer with the blank plate, or even better, a high-powered food processor such as the Cuisinart®. If you have neither, with sufficient time and patience you can use a hand blender, but take care with it as this is hard work. Put the broken-down almonds into a food processor along with all the other ingredients. Try to achieve a smooth consistency, adding a little water if necessary. Process until desired consistency is reached. Some people like chunky bits of nut to remain, while others like it smooth, or you could take half of the mixture out of the food processor while still chunky and process the rest to smoothness to create two different textures—they actually do taste a little different! Serve with green vegetables (such as lettuce, cabbage, and kale) or spread on flax crackers. This is also good as a dip and is great for taking on board a plane as it remains stable on a long flight, and is good for car trips.

Very Green Soup

(Kris Schaffer)

Serves 6–8
Prep: 25 minutes

1 cup coconut water (add more if soup becomes too thick)

1 organic cucumber with skin on

1 organic ripe avocado

2 organic green bell peppers

2 stalks organic celery hearts

4 small organic red beet tops

2 organic green onions

1 small organic green zucchini

1 handful of organic cilantro

1 handful of basil

1 teaspoon alfalfa raw honey (or to taste)

1 teaspoon minced ginger root (or to taste)

Pour the coconut water in your blender and add half of each of the veggies until completely smooth. Add more coconut water if mixture becomes too thick. Add the remaining amount of all veggies and blend until smooth. Once the veggies are blended, add a handful of each of the herbs (cilantro, basil, and ginger root). Add raw honey to taste and blend until smooth. Garnish with a couple of fresh basil leaves.

Mary's Mixed Green Salad
(Mary Schaffer)

Serves 6
Prep: 30 minutes

Salad
Handful each of baby kale,
    chard, spinach, and red
    beet tops
1 celery stalk, chopped
1 small green zucchini,
    sliced
1 red bell pepper, chopped

Special Dressing
⅓ cup cold-pressed
    flaxseed oil
Juice of 1 lemon
1 clove garlic, minced
1 teaspoon raw honey
½ inch minced ginger root
½ cup sliced, raw almonds
6 black mission figs,
    quartered

Salad
Toss ingredients together.

Special Dressing
Mix ingredients together (except almonds and figs) and pour over mixed greens. Top with ½ cup sliced raw almonds and 6 quartered black mission figs.

Robert's New Life Salad
(Robert Charles White, Ph.D.)

Prep: 20 minutes

½ cup cucumber, sliced

6 grape tomatoes

2 cups romaine lettuce

½ cup baby spinach

½ green bell pepper, chopped

½ cup yellow bell pepper, chopped

4 carrot sticks (2 inch long x ¾ inch thick)

2 pieces kale, raw or dehydrated

¼ cup sliced almonds

Combine all ingredients and drizzle with 2 tablespoons of your favorite raw dressing (optional).

Mellow Kim Chi
(Sally Bowdle)

Prep: 25 minutes
Ferment: Approximately one week (in winter, could take as long as two weeks)

1 pound napa cabbage
Bok choy, 1 head
Daikon or red radishes
2 carrots
Garlic cloves (optional)

Ginger root, grated
Chili peppers, finely
  chopped (optional)
Onions, leeks, or scallions,
  to taste
Sea salt, to taste

Make a brine by combining ¼ cup sea salt and a quart of water.

Chop cabbage and bok choy, shred daikon (or radishes) and carrots, and submerge in the brine. Let soak a few hours or overnight, until soft and salty (make another batch of brine if there isn't enough to cover).

Prepare the spices by slicing the garlic and onions (or leeks or scallions) and grating the ginger. Mix with chilies.

Drain the brine from the veggies and set aside. Make sure the veggies are salty enough; rinse if too salty or add a few teaspoons if more salt is needed.

Mix the veggies with the spices and pack into a jar or fermentation vessel. Pack down until the brine rises. Weigh down with another jar or a plastic bag filled with brine. Or just check it by tasting. Also be sure to press it down daily with clean fingers.

Let it sit (covered with a cloth) for about a week, tasting the progress every few days. Move it to the refrigerator when desired taste is reached.

Asian Slaw

(Kimberton Whole Foods, www.kimbertonwholefoods.com)

Prep: 25 minutes

¼ cup raw peanuts
1 chunk ginger (about 2 tablespoons), freshly grated
¼ cup sesame seeds
2 tablespoons olive oil
1 tablespoon sesame oil
1 tablespoon peanut oil
5 tablespoons nama shoyu
4 tablespoons raw apple cider vinegar
4 tablespoons raw honey
½ head of green cabbage, thinly sliced
¼ (or more) head of red (purple) cabbage, thinly sliced
2 carrots, julienned
1 yellow pepper, thinly sliced lengthwise

To make the dressing, first process the peanuts, ginger, and sesame seeds and set aside in a bowl. Add the liquid ingredients (olive oil, sesame oil, peanut oil, nama shoyu, apple cider vinegar, and raw honey) and stir.

For the salad, toss all sliced ingredients (cabbages, carrots, and yellow pepper) into a huge bowl and pour on the sauce and mix well.

For a lighter salad, use less dressing or more cabbage.

Note: You can use another sweetener, such as agave, if honey doesn't sit well with you. You can also use all olive oil instead of the varied oils suggested here.

Fermented Italian Green Beans

(Scott Zukay)

These are delightful crudités! Enjoy by yourself, or with friends who may not understand your diet—this should be loved by all!

Prep: 20 minutes
Ferment: 2–3 weeks

1 pound fresh, raw green beans
1 clove garlic
½ teaspoon dried oregano
½ teaspoon dried basil
1 teaspoon Celtic sea salt
4 ounces Zukay Kvass, preferably Veggie Medley
Well or spring water (non-chlorinated)

Take the ends off the green beans. Depending on what you prefer, either keep the green beans whole or cut them in half. Dice the garlic clove.

In a quart mason jar, combine all the ingredients and fill until all the beans are below the surface of the water. Make sure you leave at least a 1-inch space between the lid and the top of the water, as the mixture will expand. Close fairly tightly.

Keep the jar inside a casserole dish (in case it leaks), and leave it in a warm place (70–80°F) for 2–3 weeks. It should become fizzy—if it's not fizzy after 5 days, throw it out. You can open it to check, but this is not necessary. After 3 weeks, eat and refrigerate!

Outstanding Miso Sesame Dressing & Kale Salad

(Gena at ChoosingRaw and Kimberton Whole Foods,
www.kimbertonwholefoods.com)

Prep: 25 minutes

Dressing
½ cup mellow white miso
⅓ cup agave nectar
½ cup tahini (raw is
    preferable, but roasted
    is fine)
3–4 tablespoons tamari
½ inch fresh ginger,
    chopped (or ½
    teaspoon dry)
1¼ cups water

Salad
1 bunch curly kale
1 large beefsteak tomato,
    chopped
1 large bell pepper (or 2
    small), chopped

Dressing
Blend all ingredients on high in a Vitamix® high-speed blender.
Add more water if the mixture is too thick.

Salad
De-stem, chop, and wash kale well. Add about ⅓–½ cup of the
miso dressing to the kale. Using your hands, "massage" dressing
into salad, until it's a little wilted in texture. Add tomatoes and peppers, toss, and serve.

Thai Tomato Salad

(Kimberton Whole Foods, www.kimbertonwholefoods.com)

Prep: 25 minutes

Salad
9 campari tomatoes, diced
4 pickling cucumbers (or 1
    large English), chopped
1 red bell pepper, chopped
1 yellow pepper, chopped
½ red or yellow onion,
    diced
1 avocado, chopped
1 handful of freshly
    chopped cilantro

Dressing
¼ cup lime juice
2 tablespoons sesame oil
1½ tablespoons tamari
    (reduced sodium)
1 teaspoon miso
1 packet stevia
½ teaspoon red chili paste
    (1 teaspoon if you
    prefer more spice)

Salad
Combine all ingredients together in a bowl, set aside.

Dressing
Whisk all ingredients together and pour over salad. Serve immediately, or let marinate in refrigerator.

Stuffed Peppers

(Kimberton Whole Foods, www.kimbertonwholefoods.com)

Prep: 15 minutes

3 bell peppers
1 avocado
1 tomato
1 carrot
1 bunch of parsley
Chili pepper

In a food processor, place one bell pepper, avocado, tomato, and carrot. Process until it forms a purée. Add the parsley and chili as desired. Cut the remaining two bell peppers in half and pour the mixture inside the peppers. Serve with a green salad.

Creamy Cucumber Soup

(Kimberton Whole Foods, www.kimbertonwholefoods.com)

Prep: 25 minutes

26 ounces cucumber juice
Meat from one mature coconut
5 marigold flowers
1 seeded cherry bomb pepper
1 tablespoon miso (optional)
½ English cucumber
1½ cups soaked wakame
3 chive flowers (or use chives)
Handful cilantro flowers (or other flower)

Blend the cucumber juice with the meat from one mature coconut. Take the blended mixture and use a nut milk bag to make "cucumber milk". Blend the cucumber milk with the marigolds, cherry bomb pepper, and miso (if desired). Use a spiral slicer to spiralize half of an English cucumber. Pour the cucumber milk into a medium bowl. Add 1½ cup of wakame and half of the cucumber spaghetti to the soup base. Garnish with chive flowers and cilantro flowers.

Note: To make 26 ounces of cucumber juice, juice five regular cucumbers.

Apple and Butternut Squash Raw Soup
(Kimberton Whole Foods, www.kimbertonwholefoods.com)

Soak: Pumpkin seeds, 4 hours
Prep: 25 minutes

2 apples, cored and cut
3½ ounces peeled butternut squash
½ orange, peeled
2 tablespoons lemon juice
½ red onion
1 cup almond milk
3 tablespoons pumpkin seeds, soaked
1 tablespoon sundried tarragon
2 tablespoons chopped parsley
Salt and pepper, to taste

Blend all ingredients (except the parsley) until you have obtained a smooth and creamy soup. (You may need to add up to a glass of fresh water to obtain the desired consistency.) Serve with sprinkled parsley and season with salt and pepper to taste.

Smokey Backyard Tomato Soup with Hot Red Pepper Sauce

(Chef Barbara Shevkun, Rawfully Tempting)

Prep: 30 minutes

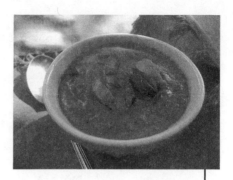

Photo courtesy of Chef Barbara Shevkun, Rawfully Tempting (www.rawfullytempting.com)

Soup

3 cups mixed garden tomatoes, roughly chopped

¼ cup sundried tomatoes, soaked

¾ cup soak water (from sundried tomatoes)

¼ cup cashews

½ small clove garlic, minced

1 red bell pepper, roughly chopped

¼ cup red onion, chopped

¼ teaspoon onion powder

⅛ teaspoon garlic powder

1 tablespoon fresh basil, chopped

1 tablespoon cilantro leaves, chopped

$\frac{1}{16}$ teaspoon smoked paprika

1 pinch cayenne

⅛ teaspoon sea salt (eliminate if sundried tomatoes are salty)

Hot Red Pepper Sauce

2 tablespoons leftover soup (from sides of blender)

3 tablespoons olive oil

½ red bell pepper

1 red chili pepper, chopped

To Serve

Sliced avocado, for garnish

Red onion, for garnish

Fresh basil or cilantro, for garnish

Pepper, to taste

Soup

Blend garden tomatoes, sundried tomatoes, and half of the soak water. Add more soak water as needed.

Add remaining ingredients and blend until creamy. Taste for seasoning and adjust as needed.

Pour into bowl, leaving about 2 tablespoons of soup in blender.

Hot Red Pepper Sauce

Scrape remains of soup into blender and add remaining ingredients. Add more oil (or water) if needed to blend.

To Serve

Pour soup into individual bowls.

Drizzle a small amount of Hot Red Pepper Sauce over soup and garnish with sliced avocado, red onion, and fresh basil or cilantro. Add fresh cracked pepper and serve.

Raw Vegetable Pasta
(Dave Scully)

Prep: 30 minutes

⅓ cup goji berries
2 zucchini squash
2 yellow summer squash
1 cup cherry or grape tomatoes
1 cup sliced shitake or reishi mushrooms
½ shallot, finely chopped
1 garlic clove, finely chopped
1 tablespoon basil, finely chopped
1 teaspoon oregano, finely chopped
1 tablespoon cold-pressed virgin olive oil
Himalayan salt and freshly ground pepper, to taste

Soak the goji berries in a small bowl of purified water for about 20 minutes, or until plump. Using a vegetable peeler, thinly shave the zucchini and yellow summer squash lengthwise into a medium or large bowl. Chop up the tomatoes, mushrooms, shallot, garlic, basil, and oregano and add them to the bowl with the slices of squash. Add the cold-pressed olive oil and season to taste with salt and pepper. Gently mix using a spatula, wooden spoon or your hands.

Add to plate and enjoy!

I Can't Believe This Isn't Pasta
(Drew Hunt)

Soak: Cashews, overnight
Prep: 35 minutes

2 cups raw cashews

Juice of 2 lemons

2 tablespoons chickpea
    miso

1 tablespoon coconut oil

2 tablespoons nutritional
    yeast (optional, not
    raw)

8 generous cups spiralized
    zucchini

2 ⅓ tablespoons sea salt

3–4 ripe tomatoes

3–4 sundried tomatoes

Cold-pressed virgin olive
    oil

1 clove garlic

Few sprigs fresh basil

¼ small red onion (or 1
    shallot)

1 teaspoon black pepper

Soak 2 cups of raw cashews overnight. Put 1¾ cups of soaked nuts into food processor with lemon juice, chickpea miso, coconut oil and 2 tablespoons nutritional yeast (optional). Process until smooth. Remove from processor and then use the processor to crumb the remaining nuts. Mix the smooth nut mixture with the crumbed nuts. Preferably set aside at room temperature for a few hours before proceeding as this will allow flavors to mature. If you don't have time, just continue to next step.

Using a spiralizer with a linguini or spaghetti blade, spiralize about 8 cups of zucchini. Using two tablespoons of sea salt toss the zucchini noodles with the salt to evenly distribute. Set to the side while making the sauce and occasionally return to hand toss the zucchini (the salt will wilt the zucchini which is intended).

Core and roughly chop several ripe tomatoes. (If tomatoes are out of season use vine-ripened roma tomatoes.) Put tomatoes in blender. Add a few sundried tomatoes, a healthy splash of cold-pressed virgin olive oil, garlic, a few sprigs of fresh basil, red onion or shallot, black pepper, and sea salt. Blend until smooth. Add olive oil to reach desired consistency.

Return to zucchini noodles. When they are limp, pliable and roughly the consistency of cooked pasta, fill the bowl with cold water, drain and repeat until the salt has been removed. (The only way to be sure the salt has been sufficiently removed is to taste the noodles.) Toss the zucchini noodles with the tomato sauce. Liberally sprinkle the nut cheese on top. Garnish generously with chopped tomatoes (different colors are nice) and chopped fresh basil or cilantro.

Baby Bella Burgers
(Dr. Karen Izzi)

Soak: Seeds, 4 hours
Prep: 25 minutes
Dehydrate: 2 hours at 105°F or until desired consistency and warmth is reached

8 ounces baby portobello mushrooms
2 cups cauliflower
2 teaspoons coconut oil
1 small onion, chopped
1 cup pumpkin seeds, soaked
1 cup sunflower seeds, soaked
½ teaspoon cayenne (optional)
Sesame seeds, as needed
Salt and pepper, to taste

In processor blend mushrooms, cauliflower, coconut oil, and onion until crumbly. Pulse in pumpkin and sunflower seeds, leaving them somewhat coarse. Shape into burgers and coat with sesame seeds. Dehydrate at 105°F for 2 hours or until "medium well." Enjoy with a raw cheese or cashew dressing and burger fixings. If you wish your burgers to be spicier, add cayenne pepper when combining the ingredients.

Mock Chicken Salad
(Dr. Karen Izzi)

Soak: Seeds, 4 hours
Prep: 20 minutes

¼ cup raw soaked sunflower seeds
1 cup raw cashews
1 medium cucumber
1 small onion
½ medium green apple, cored and seeded
1 large stalk celery
1 teaspoon dill
1 tablespoon lemon juice
4–6 sliced grapes, for garnish
Salt and pepper, to taste

Combine the above ingredients in a food processor until desired consistency. Slice grapes and serve on top as a garnish.

Happy Harvest Mushroom Tomato Salad
(Lisa Montgomery)

Prep: 20 minutes
Dehydrate: 4–6 hours at 105°F

8 ounces crimini mushrooms, sliced

8–16 ounces heirloom cherry tomatoes, quartered

2 tablespoons red onions, chopped

2 tablespoons pine nuts

2 tablespoons raisins

1 tablespoon raw honey (I use honey from my own bees)

3–4 tablespoons Austria's Pumpkin Seed Oil (enough to
    thoroughly cover all ingredients)

1 tablespoon wheat-free tamari

Sea salt and ground pepper, to taste

Combine all of the above ingredients in a bowl until thoroughly covered. Place ingredients in glass dish and place on the bottom tray of your dehydrator. Set dehydrator at 105°F and dehydrate until all of the ingredients and flavors have melded. This should take approximately 4–6 hours. (I use this method when I want my "casserole" to come out like it has been baked in a conventional oven.) Periodically, throughout the dehydrating/heating process, take the dish out and use a spoon to remix the ingredients, making sure all the ingredients are covered with the sauce so as not to get dried out.

> *I was inspired to create this recipe after having bought fresh crimini mushrooms at my local farmers market. I excitedly brought the mushrooms and then simply added what I already had at home and this is what I came up with.*

Mock Taco Meat

(Sheryll Chavarria)

Soak: Seeds, 4 hours
Prep: 15 minutes
Dehydrate: 1 hour at 105°F

2 cups sunflower seeds, soaked for 4 hours
2 tablespoons nutritional yeast
2 tablespoons cumin
2 tablespoons chili powder
Tamari, to taste

Put all ingredients into food processor and blend well. Place ingredients onto dehydrator sheets (do not use Teflex sheets, only use the mesh plastic). Dehydrate for about 1 hour at 105°F.

Healing Soup
(Kimberton Whole Foods, www.kimbertonwholefoods.com)

Prep: 20 minutes

Water of one young Thai coconut (or if unavailable, water)
1 English cucumber
2 celery ribs
½ avocado
2 large or 4 small chard leaves
3 green onions
Juice from 1 lime
Small handful of dulse seaweed (optional)
Pinch of cayenne pepper
½ bell pepper
Small handful of cilantro, mint, rosemary, or any favorite
    combo of fresh herbs
Tomato, avocado, bell pepper, green onion, seaweed, and herbs,
    for garnish

Blend coconut water, ½ English cucumber, 2 ribs celery, ½ avocado, chard leaves, 1 green onion, lime juice, seaweed, and pinch of cayenne in a powerful blender until smooth. Then add the ½ bell pepper, ½ English cucumber, 2 green onions, and the handfuls of fresh herbs. Pulse a few times until the herbs are roughly chopped. Garnish with tomato, avocado, bell pepper, green onion, torn dulse seaweed, and fresh herbs.

Trine's Seed Burgers

(Kimberton Whole Foods, www.kimbertonwholefoods.com)

Soak: Seeds, 4 hours
Prep: 25 minutes
Dehydrate: 6 hours at 105°F (or to desired doneness)

⅓ cup pumpkin seeds

⅓ cup sunflower seeds

⅓ cup ground flaxseeds (or whole)

1–2 cloves garlic

¼ cup chives, chopped

Small bunch of parsley

¼ cup yellow onion, chopped (about 1 small onion)

1 small red or orange pepper, chopped

1 stalk celery, chopped

2–3 tablespoons nama shoyu (raw soy sauce) or wheat free
    tamari

1 teaspoon cumin

Dash of cayenne pepper

Grind the pumpkin and sunflower seeds until substance reaches a meal consistency. Add to flax meal in a large bowl. (You can grind your own flax meal if you only have the seeds.) Next, place the garlic, chives, parsley, onion, pepper, and celery in a blender. (Ideally, you should chop everything up loosely beforehand as, once in the blender, you will want to set it to slowest speed and use the Vitamix® blender's plunger to mince the vegetables.) The desired result is finely chopped vegetables that are oozing a bit with liquid. If you don't have a fancy blender, you can finely chop the vegetables by hand; using a high-speed blender will help get the juices out so your burgers are easy to form, and it saves time, too.

Transfer the vegetables into the seed bowl and add the soy sauce, cumin, and cayenne. Stir until you have a burger consistency. Grab a handful of the mixture and make sure it easily sticks together. If not, you may need to add a little water. If too mushy, add more flax meal. Finally, form into patties and place in dehydrator at 105°F for as long as you like, probably at least 6 hours for a soft burger.

Sun Burgers

(Kimberton Whole Foods, www.kimbertonwholefoods.com)

Soak: Seeds, 4 hours
Prep: 20 minutes
Dehydrate: 2–3 hours at 105°F (optional)

1 cup ground sunflower seeds
½ cup ground flaxseeds
½ cup water
½ medium onion, diced
½ red bell pepper, finely chopped
¾ cup celery, finely chopped
Avocado, tomato, and alfalfa sprouts, for garnish

Process the sunflower seeds and flaxseeds well in a processor and transfer to a bowl. Mix in ½ cup water, or less, if you prefer your burgers to be dryer. Chop the onions, peppers, and celery into very small pieces and mix in by spoon. Add remaining water until desired consistency is reached for forming balls and flattening into patties. Dehydrate the patties for several hours (or less if making smaller patties), making sure they are slightly crunchy on the surface. You can even opt not to dehydrate them at all. Garnish with avocado, tomato, and alfalfa sprouts and place on a bed of lettuce. Try some raw catsup or another raw sauce with these burgers.

Cauliflower Sushi Rolls

(Kimberton Whole Foods, www.kimbertonwholefoods.com)
This is a very easy recipe but the assembly just takes a little extra time until you get the trick of rolling your own sushi.

Prep: 30 minutes

Cauliflower Rice
½ head of cauliflower
2 diced spring onions
¼ cup pine nuts
1 teaspoon tamari sauce
Juice of ½ lemon
Salt, to taste

Sushi Assembly
1 nori sheet
¼ ripe avocado, sliced
Handful of sprouts
Greens of your choice
Tamari or nama shoyu, for
    dipping

Cauliflower Rice
Pulse cauliflower until it reaches a rice-like consistency. Add the remaining ingredients and pulse again until combined. Adjust salt and tamari sauce to taste.

Sushi Assembly
Place one nori sheet shiny-side down on a sushi mat (if available). Cover bottom half of nori with cauliflower "rice." Layer on sliced avocado, sprouts, and greens. Roll sushi mat away from you and tighten roll. Seal edge with water. Slice roll into bite-size pieces with a sharp knife.

   Repeat the process until all the filling is used up. Dip in tamari or nama shoyu sauce and pop into your mouth!

Live Un-Stir-Fry with Cauliflower "Rice"

(Kimberton Whole Foods, www.kimbertonwholefoods.com)

Serves 4
Prep: 30 minutes

Vegetable Medley
2 cups chopped napa cabbage
1 cup thinly sliced red bell pepper
¾ cup raw unsalted cashews (optional)
½ cup chopped red cabbage
½ cup thinly sliced carrots
½ cup thinly sliced snow peas
¼ cup thinly sliced green onion
2 tablespoons chopped cilantro

Spicy Vegetable Dressing
½ cup sesame oil
1 fresh stalk lemongrass, outer leaves removed, finely chopped
    (optional)
3 tablespoons raw agave nectar or maple syrup
3 tablespoons nama shoyu or soy sauce
2 tablespoons umeboshi plum vinegar or raw apple cider
    vinegar
1½-inch piece peeled fresh ginger
1 tablespoon dehydrated onion flakes
1 tablespoon tamarind paste (optional)
1 tablespoon grated lime zest
1 clove garlic, peeled
1 teaspoon minced Thai or jalapeño chili
1 small kaffir lime leaf

Cauliflower Rice
4 cups cauliflower florets
½ cup macadamia or pine nuts
1 tablespoon dehydrated onion flakes
½ teaspoon sea salt
½ teaspoon garlic powder

Vegetable Medley
Combine all ingredients in large bowl.

Spicy Vegetable Dressing
Place all ingredients in blender or food processor, and blend until creamy. Add to vegetable medley, and toss well.

Cauliflower Rice
Place all ingredients in food processor, and pulse-chop to rice-like consistency. Serve topped with the vegetable medley.

Raw Vegan Lasagna Vegetable Stacks

(Kimberton Whole Foods, www.kimbertonwholefoods.com)
Prep: 45–60 minutes

Lasagna Sheets
2 large zucchinis
3 yellow squash or yellow
  zucchini
6 large tomatoes, sliced
Basil leaves
Olive oil
Cherry tomatoes (optional)
Gomasio (optional)

Raw Tomato Sauce
2 cups sundried tomatoes
1 cup chopped tomatoes (2
  medium tomatoes)
¼ cup cold-pressed extra-
  virgin olive oil
2 teaspoons fresh garlic
¾ teaspoon Celtic sea salt
1 teaspoon dried basil
¼ teaspoon red pepper
  flakes

Basil Pesto
5 cups tightly packed fresh
  basil leaves
1½ cups raw macadamias,
  soaked (optional)
½ cup olive oil
1½ teaspoon Celtic sea salt
2 tablespoons lemon zest
3 tablespoons lemon juice
6 tablespoons garlic

Macadamia Ricotta
2 cups raw macadamias,
  soaked (optional)
¾ cup–1 cup filtered water
  for desired consistency
2 tablespoons fresh lime
  juice
2 tablespoons finely
  chopped serrano chili
  (chillier to taste)
1 tablespoon finely minced
  fresh garlic
2 teaspoons yellow mustard
  powder
½ teaspoon Celtic sea salt
¼ cup finely chopped
  cilantro/coriander

Lasagna Sheets

Hold each zucchini and, using vegetable peeler (or mandolin), peel off large thin strips of the zucchini. Peel the yellow squash and cut the tomatoes into ¼-inch or ½-inch thick slices. Set aside on layers of paper towel to remove any excess liquid while you make the sauces.

Raw Tomato Sauce

Throw all the ingredients in a food processor and pulse until well combined. Season to taste. (You want this sauce to be mild in order to blend with the pesto and the ricotta.)

Basil Pesto

Throw all the ingredients in a food processor and pulse until well combined.

Macadamia Ricotta

Throw all of the ingredients (except cilantro) into a food processor and pulse until well combined and fluffy. Stir through the chopped cilantro.

To assemble, lay out six large plates. Lay three slices of zucchini side by side to make a wide rectangle lasagna sheet base. Spread some red sauce on top of each base. Lay three slices of yellow squash or zucchini on top of the sauce. Place two tomato slices on top of the ricotta. Now place three more pieces of zucchini to make another sheet of pasta. Spread a layer of green pesto and top with two more pieces of tomato. Garnish with large fresh basil leaves and drizzle the whole plate with a bit of olive oil. You could also surround the lasagna with some chopped cherry tomatoes tossed in olive oil or garnish with some gomasio.

Raw Thai Curry

(Kimberton Whole Foods, www.kimbertonwholefoods.com)

Prep: 20 minutes

2 avocados
2 (dried) lime leaves
¼–½ fresh chili
1 teaspoon lime juice
¾ inch lemongrass stem
¾ inch cube fresh ginger
½ loosely packed cup fresh coriander (cilantro)
½–1 cup pure water (or as needed for desired consistency)
½ tablespoon curry powder

Simply blend all ingredients together, either in a blender or food processor until everything is fully blended. Taste test. Add more water if you'd like it runnier. Add more lemongrass and a tomato, and/or avocado if it's too hot.

DINNER

Sprouted Kamut Sushi
(Kimberton Whole Foods, www.kimbertonwholefoods.com)

Sprout: 3 days
Prep: 30 minutes

1 portobello mushroom
3 tablespoons nami shoyu, divided
2 tablespoons olive oil
2 cups sprouted kamut
1 tablespoon sesame oil
2 carrots
½ cucumber
1 avocado
Nori sheets
Sunflower sprouts, as needed to fill out sushi roll

Cut the portobello mushroom into slices about ¼- to ½-inch thick. Toss with 2 tablespoons nama shoyu and 2 tablespoons oil and let sit for at least 30 minutes. Process the kamut, remaining 2 tablespoons nama shoyu, and sesame oil in a food processor until the kamut starts to break apart. Set aside. Slice carrots and cucumber into match stick–sized pieces. Slice the avocado into ¼ inch pieces. Set aside. Lay a nori sheet on a sushi mat (if available). Spread half the sheet with the kamut mixture. Place the avocado, carrots, cucumber, sunflower sprouts, and mushrooms on top of the kamut. Using the mat, carefully and tightly roll the seaweed into a sushi roll. Cut with a serrated knife.

Basic Kale Salad

(Lisa Montgomery)

Prep: 10 minutes

2 bunches kale
1 tablespoon lemon juice
2 tablespoons cold-pressed olive oil (or Austria's Finest
    Naturally® Pumpkin Seed Oil)
Sea salt, to taste

Remove the kale leaves from stems. Rip the leaves into bite size pieces or cut them in chiffonade style to make them look more attractive. Massage the lemon juice, olive oil, and salt into the kale to break it down.

You can also add whatever your heart desires such as sundried tomatoes, fresh diced or sliced tomatoes, olives, avocados, red peppers, or onions.

Basic Spring Mix Salad

(Lisa Montgomery)

This is such an obvious salad to make, but sometimes life is just so busy that you need to keep it simple and uncomplicated.

Prep: 5 minutes

Spring Mix

Assorted vegetables (such as tomatoes, onion, and avocado)

Dressing of your choice (or Austria's Finest Naturally® Pumpkin Seed Oil)

Simply throw a handful of spring mix into a bowl and add your favorite dressing (or a little Austria's Finest Naturally® Pumpkin Seed Oil). You can just eat the simple greens or you can add your favorite vegetables.

Chili Con Amore
(Sheryll Chavarria)

Prep: 30 minutes
Dehydrate: Several hours at 105°F (optional)

1 cup zucchini, chopped
1 large portobello mushroom, chopped
2 cups corn, cut off the cob
1 cup fresh tomatoes, chopped
½ red bell pepper, chopped fine
½ cup onion, chopped fine
1 tablespoon cumin powder
1 tablespoon chili powder
2 tablespoons tamari
2 cloves garlic
3 tablespoons olive oil
1 red bell pepper, chopped coarsely
1 cup tomato, chopped coarsely
1 cup sundried tomatoes

Soak sundried tomatoes in water, keeping approximately 1 cup soaking water.

Mix the zucchini, mushroom, corn, tomatoes, bell pepper, and onion in a bowl and set aside. Blend remaining ingredients. Add reserved soaking water to blended ingredients as needed if the mixture is too dry. (Do not pour all in at once.) Mix into bowl with chopped vegetables. Serve. This can also be warmed in a dehydrator for several hours at 105°F to allow the flavors to meld.

Truly Raw Coleslaw (and Mayonnaise)
(Kimberton Whole Foods, www.kimbertonwholefoods.com)

Prep: 25 minutes

Mayonnaise
1 cup water
1 cup macadamia nuts
1 cup pine nuts
1½ cups cashew nuts
½ teaspoon crystal salt
1 tablespoon apple cider vinegar
2 tablespoons lemon juice

Slaw
4 large carrots, chopped
1 small onion, chopped
1 small cabbage, chopped or shredded

Mayonnaise
Combine all ingredients in a Vitamix® high-speed blender or food processor until thoroughly blended and set aside.

Slaw
Chop the carrots, onion, and cabbage into fairly small pieces and place in a food processor. Pulse until all ingredients are well combined and become the perfect slaw shape and size. Pour them into a large bowl and set aside for mixing. Rinse the food processor then add the mayonnaise ingredients. Be sure to mix very well adding more water if needed or desired. When fully blended, pour three quarters of the mayonnaise on top of the slaw and mix with a large spoon until the salad mixture is thoroughly coated. If you like more coverage, add more mayonnaise.

This mayonnaise recipe also makes a great dressing, dip, or filling for nori rolls and wraps whether they be collard leaves or flax wraps.

The refrigerator life span of mayonnaise is 5–7 days. The coleslaw mixture with mayonnaise is good for three or four days in the refrigerator (don't worry, you'll eat it by then).

Sauerkraut

(Lisa Montgomery)

Prep: 30 minutes
Ferment: 3–5 days in summer, up to 2 weeks in winter

Red and green cabbages
Radishes
Daikon
Onion
Herbs such as parsley, dill, and scallions, to taste (I personally
    throw in a few handfuls)
Spiralized vegetables such as beets, yellow squash, yams, and
    zucchini
Sea salt

Shred all vegetables. Combine all ingredients in a bowl. For every
quart of ingredients, add a tablespoon of sea salt. Mix it together,
place in a canning jar, and pack it tightly leaving approximately 1
inch of space at the top of the jar (it is important to leave this space
because when you keep packing down the vegetables, the liquid
will rise).

Cover it with two pieces of cheesecloth and use a rubber band
or the ring for the canning jar to hold the cheesecloth in place.
Set the jar on your countertop. Twice a day, take off the ring and
cheesecloth and with clean hands keep pushing down on the vegetables (the liquid continues to rise to the top and will eventually
evaporate).

In the summer, the sauerkraut will ferment in 3–7 days depending on your local temperature. In the winter, it will take a few
weeks. Once it has fermented, place the lid on the canning jar and
store it in your refrigerator.

This is a basic and easy sauerkraut recipe that I learned from David Siller during my permaculture class with Melissa Miles at Permanent Future. The amounts for all ingredients can be adjusted to taste.

Fermented food is good for the gut and acts as a probiotic, as well as tasting great. When making sauerkraut this way, you can toss in any shredding ingredients from other raw dishes and any homegrown vegetables.

I tend to eat sauerkraut on a bed of greens with a pâté. I also spread it on a nori sheet with cut up produce like onions, carrots, cucumber, and slices of avocado. If you like wraps, you can spread the sauerkraut on flax or collard leaves and fill with a pâté and cut up vegetables. Add it to mung bean sprouts or sea kelp noodles and sauce and it becomes a complete meal!

Banana Chip Addiction

(Dr. Karen Izzi)

Makes about 15 chips
Prep: 15 minutes
Dehydrate: 24 hours or until crispy, at 110°F

3–4 medium bananas
2 tablespoons agave syrup
½ cup sesame seeds

Cut bananas in half then cut into slices, dipping each slice in the agave syrup. Sprinkle sesame seeds on each slice. Place on dehydrator shelf and dehydrate at 110°F for 24 hours or until crispy. Remove from mat and enjoy.

Raw Corn Chips

(Dr. Karen Izzi)

Prep: 20 minutes
Dehydrate: 8 hours or until crispy, at 100°F

6 ears fresh corn, removed from the cob
½ cup ground flaxseeds
1 small onion, diced
½ teaspoon salt
½ teaspoon pepper
½ teaspoon garlic salt

Combine ingredients in a food processor using the S blade until batter is thoroughly combined. Place mixture on non-stick dehydrator sheet.

Flatten on sheet and dehydrate for 8 hours at 100°F or until crispy.

Brazil Nut Pâté

(Kimberton Whole Foods, www.kimbertonwholefoods.com)

Prep: 10 minutes

1 cup Brazil nuts
1 clove garlic
1-inch fresh ginger
Sea salt, to taste

Place all ingredients into a high-speed blender or food processor, adding a little water if needed. Process until desired consistency is reached. This goes perfectly with crudités.

Spur of the Moment Trail Mix

(Lisa Montgomery)

One day, I needed to make a quick trail mix for some extra energy after a kick butt exercise session. I always have on hand jars of raw nuts that I have soaked, dehydrated, and stored in sealed canning jars, so I was able to easily create this tasty treat.

Soak: Seeds, 4 hours
        Almonds, 8 hours
Prep: 5 minutes

1 cup soaked and dehydrated Austria's Finest Naturally® Pumpkin Seeds

1 cup raw almonds

1 cup raw walnuts

1 cup raw sesame seeds

Sea salt and garlic powder, to taste

Toss the nuts, seeds, and spices together and store in a sealed container.

You can add any spices you like to this mixture, including dried coconut shavings, raisins, or any other assorted dried fruits. Make this recipe your own and have fun with it!

Sweet & Gooey Trail Mix Cookies
(Lisa Montgomery)

Soak: Nuts, 8 hours
Prep: 20 minutes
Dehydrate: Until warm, at 105°F

1 cup raw almonds, soaked and dried
1 cup raw walnuts, soaked and dried
½–1 cup dried fruit (such as goji berries, blueberries, cherries, or cranberries)
1–1½ cups raw cacao nibs
½ cup shredded coconut
1 tablespoon raw honey
1 teaspoon cinnamon
1 teaspoon coconut butter

Combine all ingredients and dehydrate at 105°F until warm.

Fermented Garlic Carrot Sticks
Sally Bowdle

Prep: 20 minutes
Ferment: 4 weeks

¾ pound fresh, raw carrots
1 clove garlic (or to taste)
1 teaspoon Celtic sea salt
4 ounces Zukay Kvass, preferably Veggie Medley or
    Carrot Ginger
Well or spring water (non-chlorinated)

Julienne the carrots into 3-inch strips (don't bother peeling, especially if they're farm fresh). Slice the garlic clove into thin strips (you can also choose to add a little more garlic, or even leave it out altogether).

In a quart mason jar, combine all the ingredients, and fill until the carrots are below the surface of the water. Close fairly tightly, making sure to leave at least 1 inch of space between the lid and the top of the water as the mixture will expand.

Keep the jar inside a casserole dish (in case it leaks), and leave it in a warm place (70–80°F) for 4–6 weeks. The mixture should become fizzy; if it's not fizzy after 5 days, throw it out. You can open the jar if you want, but it's not necessary. After 4 weeks, eat and refrigerate!

This is another wonderful crudités, and is especially loved by children. It makes a magnificent, super-healthy addition to any veggie plate!

Kat's Kale Chips
(Sheryll Chavarria)

Soak: 2 hours
Prep: 20 minutes
Dehydrate: 4–6 hours at 105°F (or until crispy)

1 cup soaked cashews
2 cloves garlic, pressed
¼ cup nutritional yeast
½ tablespoon cumin
½ tablespoon chili powder
½ teaspoon oregano
⅓ cup water
2 tablespoons olive oil
3 bunches kale
¼–½ cup tamari

Put cashews and garlic in food processor. Add all remaining ingredients (except the kale and tamari) and process until blended well.

Remove stems from kale and cut into large pieces. Put kale into a large bowl with blended ingredients and then brush tamari over kale. Put into dehydrator at 105°F for 4–6 hours (or until crispy).

Spicy BBQ Zucchini Chips
(Chef Barbara Shevkun, Rawfully Tempting)

Soak: Seeds, 2 hours
Prep: 30 minutes
Dehydrate: 2 hours at 110°F, flip and dehydrate for another 2–3 hours, plus another 12–15 hours or until crispy

1 cup filtered water

2 tablespoons lemon juice

2 tablespoons olive oil

3 tablespoons sunflower seeds, soaked 2 hours

1 tablespoon chia seeds

4 sundried tomatoes, soaked and chopped

1 tablespoon onion powder

2 tablespoons maple syrup (grade B or your favorite sweetener)

1½ teaspoons cilantro, dried

1 teaspoon basil, dried

¾ teaspoon paprika

¼ teaspoon garlic powder

¼ teaspoon hot red chili powder (very spicy)

⅛ teaspoon chili powder

½ teaspoon sea salt

⅛ teaspoon cayenne (optional)

½ teaspoon liquid smoke (optional, but really gives the BBQ authentic flavor)*
Hemp or chia seeds, to garnish (optional)

Chips
4-5 zucchinis

BBQ Sauce
Add all ingredients to blender and mix until sunflower seeds and tomatoes are completely processed. Scrape down sides of blender if needed and continue to blend until well mixed.

Chips
Wash and peel (or partially peel) zucchini and slice thinly using a sharp knife, peeler, or mandolin (a mandolin or box grater work

best to get the thinnest slice, but be careful not to make them too thin, or they will fall apart).

Transfer zucchini to a large mixing bowl. Pour half of the batter over zucchini and gently mix. Coat each slice well, adding more batter as needed. (Save some to re-coat when you flip chips over). Place on non-stick dehydrator trays so that chips are lying flat and not touching each other. Dehydrate at 110°F for about 2 hours.

Peel slices up from sheet and carefully turn over. Re-coat with batter as needed. Dehydrate for 2–3 hours.

Carefully remove and transfer chips to mesh dehydrator tray and continue to dehydrate 12–15 hours (depending on humidity and thickness of chips), until dry and crunchy. Depending upon humidity, they may stay a little chewy, but will still fabulously melt in your mouth!

Instead of liquid smoke, try using smoked paprika or smoked sundried tomatoes.

You can garnish the chips with sprouted quinoa or hemp seed. Sprouted quinoa is a staple in our home; I keep a jar of them in the freezer to toss on salads or grind into flour. I prefer the chips with the hemp seed, but try both and see which you like best.

For those of you who like a thicker chip (less reminiscent of a potato chip) and want to add either hemp seed or sprouted/dehydrated quinoa, just cut it thicker, leave all of the skin, and use the garnish as directed.

If you don't have a dehydrator, these can be baked (though I have not yet tried this method). Check after 1 hour for desired crispiness. Preheat oven to 350°F and then turn off the oven. Place chips on tray for l hour. Flip and let dry for balance. You'll have to keep checking to make sure they do not burn.

A friend gave us some overgrown zucchinis. Since large zucchinis do not spiralize well, we thought about making some "potato" chips. These are so incredibly reminiscent of BBQ potato chips, I can't believe it! Warning: they are very spicy, so cut down on the hot red chili powder and cayenne if you want a tamer version.

Summer Squash Slaw

(Dr. Karen Izzi)

Serves 4
Prep: 25 minutes

1 large yellow squash, shredded or spiraled
1 large carrot, shredded
1 small onion, chopped
2 small radishes, sliced
1 large avocado, cut in 1-inch chunks
6 large mushrooms, sliced
½ cup raw soaked almonds, sliced
Juice of ½ medium lemon

Combine all ingredients (except lemon juice) in a large bowl, and then stir in lemon juice. Put in refrigerator for 30 minutes and serve cold.

Carrot and Coconut Slaw

(Dr. Karen Izzi)

Prep: 20 minutes

2 cups shredded cabbage

8–10 shredded medium carrots

1 medium onion chopped

1 tablespoon ginger

1 clove fresh garlic, minced

2 tablespoons lemon juice

½ cup raw shredded coconut

Combine ingredients in large bowl. Toss, serve, and eat.

Creamy Green Garlic & Dill Dressing

(Chef Barbara Shevkun, Rawfully Tempting)

Prep: 15 minutes

½ cup cashews

6 tablespoons olive oil

1–2 large cloves garlic, minced

2 tablespoons fresh dill, chopped

½ cup water (add more if needed)

2 tablespoons horseradish, grated (optional)

2 teaspoons raw honey or liquid sweetener

⅛ teaspoon Himalayan sea salt

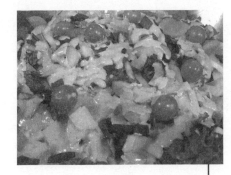

Photo courtesy of Chef Barbara Shevkun, Rawfully Tempting (www.rawfullytempting.com)

Blend all ingredients until creamy. Drizzle over salad or serve as a dip for vegetables.

Red Pepper Cheeze Sauce
(Linda Cooper)

Soak: Almonds and walnuts, 8 hours
Cashews, 1–2 hours
Prep: 20 minutes

Juice of 4–5 lemons
⅔ cup raw soaked almonds
⅔ cup raw soaked cashews or walnuts
1 teaspoon sea salt
¾–1 teaspoon turmeric
Water (only if needed to blend)
1 red bell pepper, seeded and roughly chopped
1 tablespoon nutritional yeast (optional, not raw)
¼–½ cup cold-pressed extra-virgin olive oil

Blend all ingredients (except olive oil) in a Vitamix® high-speed blender until smooth. Slowly drizzle in the olive oil to thicken the sauce (if sauce is still too thin, drop in a couple more almonds or cashews until desired consistency is reached).

This sauce is super versatile! You can cover your kale chips with this sauce before dehydrating for a cheesy chip, or spread this on top of a pizza, zucchini noodles, or raw crackers. Delicious!

Raw Pesto Sauce

(Linda Cooper)
Enjoy this pesto on raw pasta, crackers, or just about anything!

Soak: Nuts, 4 hours
Prep: 15 minutes

2 cups basil leaves
2 cups baby spinach
1 cup raw soaked walnuts
½ cup lemon juice
½–1 cup cold-pressed extra-virgin olive oil
Salt and pepper, to taste

Blend all ingredients (except olive oil) in a Vitamix® high-speed blender or food processor until everything is well combined. Slowly drizzle in the olive oil to thicken the sauce and reach desired consistency.

Basil can be expensive, especially when it's out of season. Adding equal parts spinach to basil in this recipe is a great way to get more bang for your buck.

Creamy Peppercorn Ranch Dressing

(Kimberton Whole Foods, www.kimbertonwholefoods.com)

Makes 2¼ cups
Prep: 15 minutes

⅓ cup water
⅓ cup lemon juice
⅔ cup hemp seed
5 cloves garlic
2 teaspoons whole black peppercorns
1 teaspoon Himalayan salt
1 cup cold-pressed olive oil

Place all ingredients (except olive oil) in a high-powered blender. Blend from low to high speed until smooth. With the blender running on low, pour in the olive oil to emulsify. Gradually turn up the power until ingredients are combined. The result should be very thick, creamy, and delicious. Add as a topping to any variety of fantastic fresh veggies!

Fast Alfredo Sauce

(Kimberton Whole Foods, www.kimbertonwholefoods.com)

Serves 2–3
Prep: 15–20 minutes

1 cup water (the original recipe called for soy milk)

⅓ cup raw cashews (or a wee bit more to compensate for soy milk omission)

¼ cup nutritional yeast

3 tablespoons tamari or nama shoyu

2 tablespoons margarine (in the original recipe; I simply omit this)

1 tablespoon tahini

1 tablespoon lemon juice

2 teaspoons mustard (ideally Dijon)

½ teaspoon paprika

1 pinch nutmeg

2–4 cloves garlic

Black pepper, to taste

Add all the ingredients to a blender and blend until smooth. Pour over spiralized zucchini noodles.

The cooked version (in addition to the soy milk mentioned): Drain the pasta and return it to the hot empty pan. Pour the sauce over, place on medium heat, and stir until heated through. Serve with lots of fresh cracked black pepper, and steamed broccoli, if desired.

The whole sauce is made in a blender, so the faster you can toss ingredients into a blender, the faster it's done. This also makes it super easy for additions. Try adding red peppers, for instance.

Raw Catsup

(Kimberton Whole Foods, www.kimbertonwholefoods.com)

Prep: 10 minutes

1 tomato, diced (about 1½ cups)
3 tablespoons pitted dates
¼ cup extra-virgin olive oil
1 teaspoon sea salt
1 tablespoon apple cider vinegar
½ cup sundried tomatoes

Blend fresh tomato, dates, olive oil, salt, and vinegar until smooth. If your food blender or processor is not high speed or you want a smooth texture or both, pre-soak and chop the dates well. Add the sundried tomatoes last, and blend until thick and well mixed.

I personally like this recipe with even less vinegar, as the sundried tomatoes already add a strong bite. Also, I recommend presoaking the sundried tomatoes. If yours were bought pre-packed in oil, you might want to soak them to remove the oil, unless you are certain of the quality of the soak oil (there may be table salt and other additives in the oil). In either case, finely chopping the sundried tomatoes might help with the blending if you have a weaker mixing device.

Creamy Lemon, Dill & Garlic Salad Dressing/Dip

(Kimberton Whole Foods, www.kimbertonwholefoods.com)

Serves 4
Prep: 15 minutes

½ cup raw cashews, soaked and drained
Juice from half a lemon
1½ tablespoons dill weed (or to taste)
1 clove garlic (or 2 cloves for more garlic flavor)
2 tablespoons olive oil
1 tablespoon flax or hemp oil
½ teaspoon sea salt (or to taste)
¼ cup water

Toss all ingredients into a food processor and process until smooth and creamy. Toss with your favorite salad or serve as a dip with your favorite raw crackers or veggies.

Your taste buds will tingle with this delicious dressing that is full of flavor. It is tangy and creamy and can be used as either a dressing for salads or as a dip for crudités.

Papaya-Banana Swirl Ice Cream

(Chef Barbara Shevkun, Rawfully Tempting)

Prep: 25 minutes

2 frozen bananas
½ frozen papaya, cut into
    chunks
¼ cup shredded coconut
    (for topping)
1 tablespoon hemp seed
    (for topping)
Almond cream (optional,
    see below)

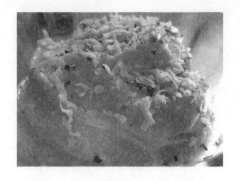

Photo courtesy of Chef Barbara Shevkun, Rawfully Tempting (www.rawfullytempting.com)

Using your juicer's blank plate, press the frozen fruit through the juicer. (If you are using a blender, cut the frozen fruit into chunks and add to blender.) You may have to add some coconut water or liquid to get it to blend. If it becomes too thin, pour into a casserole dish or bowl and chill. Cut in chunks and run through blender or food processor again. It's a bit of work, but still very yummy! Alternate ingredients though the juicer: frozen fruit, frozen bananas, frozen almond cream. The amounts are up to you, but this gives you a wonderful, creamy ice cream. Top with shredded coconut and hemp seed.

Note: If you don't have a juicer, follow the directions in the box on the next page.

Usually when I make ice cream in the blender, I'll add other ingredients like Sunflower Lecithin and Irish Moss Paste which helps to emulsify the mixture.

Almond Cream

Soak 1 cup of almonds overnight and then drain. Blend the almonds with 3 cups water. If using a blank plate don't strain. Otherwise, strain nut cream through a screen, cheesecloth, or nut milk bag. Sweeten with your favorite liquid sweetener (such as grade B maple syrup, optional). Freeze cream in silicone molds or ice cube trays.

Note: I always soak a lot of almonds, drain, then dehydrate them and store in a large canning jar so that I always have almonds ready to go.

For those of you without a juicer that has a blank plate, fret not—you can have ice cream too. Here are several options:

1. *Blend the ingredients together and freeze. Run through blender or food processor.*
2. *Blend almond cream, frozen papaya, and frozen bananas and run through an ice cream maker until desired consistency is reached.*
3. *Freezing the mixture, stirring every hour until it reaches the consistency of soft serve ice cream. If it gets too hard, let it soften a bit and serve.*
4. *Use a Yonanas® machine (www.yonanas.com). I've never tried it, but it looks fabulous!*

Pecan Cake
(Dawn Light)

Makes two 6-inch cakes
Prep: 15 minute plus refrigeration

½ cup dates (about 8)
1¼ cups pecans

Pit dates and, if they're hard, soak until soft but not mushy. Chop pecans in food processor. Remove pecans from processor. Blend dates until chopped into small pieces. Mix dates and chopped pecans thoroughly.

Form into the shape of two 6-inch cakes (or any other shapes you want) and chill in the refrigerator.

After the cakes are solid you can frost them individually if you like or fill, layer, and frost them as one cake. Lemon frosting and chocolate frosting make this cake even nicer!

Store in the refrigerator.

Note: The more your dates and pecans are chopped, the denser your cake will be.

Lemon Frosting
(Dawn Light)
This recipe will frost and fill a 6-inch two-layer cake

Prep: 10 minutes

1¾ cups cashews
⅓ cup lemon juice
2 teaspoons lemon pulp (optional)
½ cup raw honey

Blend cashews and lemon juice with pulp (pulp is optional) until it turns into a liquid.

Add honey while food processor is running. Blend thoroughly until the mixture becomes a smooth liquid. Scrape the sides of the bowl frequently.

　　To frost, simply spread the frosting on the cake.

　　If using as a cake filling, spread frosting on top of one cake layer and place the second cake layer on top before frosting the entire cake.

Raw Key Lime Pudding
Rhonda Malkmus

Prep: 20 minutes

3 medium avocados, peeled and pitted
1 ripe banana
¾ cup fresh or frozen mango pieces
1 cup fresh lime juice (about 5 limes)
1 teaspoon lime zest
½ cup raw unfiltered honey or agave nectar
¼ cup organic coconut oil
¼ fresh vanilla bean or 1½ teaspoon pure vanilla
½ teaspoon Celtic or Himalayan salt

Place all ingredients into Vitamix® high-speed blender or other powerful blender and process until smooth and creamy.

Cheesecake Stuffed Strawberries

(Dr. Karen Izzi)

Prep: 20 minutes

1 cup cashews
¼ cup honey
2 tablespoons almond milk
1 teaspoon vanilla
Dash of cinnamon
1 pound strawberries
Raw cocoa or chocolate shavings

Blend cashews, honey, almond milk, vanilla, and cinnamon in a high-powered blender until whipped smooth.

Wash and remove stems of strawberries, hollowing out a bit of the berry.

Stuff the strawberries with cheese filling using a pastry bag or a plastic bag cut at the corner.

Drizzle with raw cocoa or shavings of chocolate. Refrigerate until ready to eat.

Raw Tart Crust
(Dr. Karen Izzi)

Soak: Almonds, 8 hours
Prep: 20 minutes

1 cup almonds, soaked
1 cup cashews
1 cup pitted dates
½ teaspoon vanilla extract
Pinch of salt

Combine all ingredients in a food processor until smooth. Put crust in pie plate and add your favorite filling such as fresh strawberries or blueberries. You can also sprinkle the fruit with raw honey, cinnamon, or lemon juice (or a combination of all three).

The Best Raw Cookie

(Dr. Karen Izzi)

Soak: Hazelnuts, 6 hours
Prep: 25 minutes
Dehydrate: 9 hours at 105°F (optional)

¼ cup sunflower oil

5 cups raw oats

2 cups raisins

1 cup raw chunky peanut butter

½ cup flaxseeds

1 cup hazelnuts, soaked

1 cup chopped walnuts

1 cup chopped dried apricots

1 tablespoon vanilla

¾ cup agave syrup

Combine ingredients in a food processor until mixture is totally combined. Form into 1-inch balls then slightly flatten with a wooden spoon or form into desired shape. You can either eat these cookies raw or dehydrate on a Teflex sheet at 105°F for 9 hours or until desired consistency is reached. Flip the cookie after 4 hours and remove Teflex sheet. These are great for fighting sweet-tooth cravings.

Mango Tango Cake
(Linda Cooper)

Soak: Nuts, 8 hours
Prep: 45–60 minutes

Crust
1 cup raw soaked almonds
1 cup raw soaked walnuts, pecans, or cashews
1 cup unsweetened, dried coconut shreds
¼ teaspoon sea salt
¼ cup sweetener of choice (agave nectar, raw honey, or coconut nectar)
¼ cup coconut butter

Filling
3 cups raw soaked cashews
2 cups mango
1½ cups orange juice
⅓ cup lemon juice
⅓ cup grade B maple syrup (not a raw product)
¾ cup sweetener of choice (agave, raw honey, or coconut nectar)
Vanilla beans of 1 vanilla pod
⅛ teaspoon sea salt
1½ cups coconut oil, melted
1 tablespoon sunflower lecithin

Optional Crumb Topping
Reserved crust
½ cup freeze-dried mangoes

Crust

Combine all dry ingredients in a food processor until a sand-like texture is reached. Add sweetener and coconut butter to mixture and blend again until all ingredients are well incorporated. Crust should stick together when pressed. Add ¾ of the crust to a lined, 10-inch springform pan. Reserve ¼ of crust for crumb topping (optional). Press down and smooth crust in pan with a tamper or the back of a spoon until the entire bottom of the pan is covered. Set aside in freezer.

Note: Be careful to not over mix; the nuts will eventually release their oils and make nut butter!

Filling

Combine all ingredients (except coconut oil and sunflower lecithin) in a high-speed blender. Blend until a smooth texture is reached; there should be no grit left in the mixture. Add the coconut oil and sunflower lecithin to blender. Combine on high speed until all ingredients are completely incorporated, while being careful not to overheat the mixture. Pour all contents of the blender into the crust-lined springform pan. Add optional crumb topping and freeze overnight for a delicious cake (but see below first)!

Optional Crumb Topping

Process ingredients together in a food processor until a crumbly texture is achieved. Add crumbs to the top of your cake before freezing.

Carrot/Apple Ginger Cookies
(Mary Schaffer)

Soak: Groats, 6–8 hours
Prep: 30 minutes
Dehydrate: 10–12 hours at 105°F

⅓ cup buckwheat groats, soaked 6 to 8 hours
1 cup organic carrot pulp (see note below)
1 cup apple pulp (see note below)
2 teaspoons freshly minced ginger
1 teaspoon cinnamon
½ cup raw coconut crystals
⅓ cup organic raisins
½ cup chopped raw nuts (such as pecans, cashews, or almonds)
¼ cup cold-pressed organic olive oil

Mix all ingredients in a medium size bowl and shape into cookies about the size of a ginger snap. Put them in a dehydrator overnight, about 10–12 hours, at 105°F.

If you don't have carrot pulp or apple pulp, you can substitute with chopped carrots and apples.

Maple Pecan Ice Cream

(Kimberton Whole Foods, www.kimbertonwholefoods.com)

Prep: 25 minutes
Freeze: 6 hours or overnight

3 ripe bananas
½ cup raw almond butter
½ cup raw tahini (sesame butter)
¾ cup dark agave nectar
¼ cup raw honey
1 teaspoon vanilla extract
1 tablespoon ground cinnamon
1 cup pecans, chopped (optional)

Combine all ingredients (except the pecans) in a food processor. Process until creamy. Stir in pecans. Freeze in an airtight container for 6 hours or overnight.

Banoffe Pie

(Kimberton Whole Foods, www.kimbertonwholefoods.com)

Prep: 30–40 minutes

Base
4 cups oat groats, blended
   to a fine powder
¾ cup maple syrup
1 tablespoon almond
   butter
Pinch of salt
3–4 bananas, sliced

Toffee
1 cup almond butter
1 cup maple syrup
Pinch of salt

Cream Topping
5 bananas
1 cup almond butter
Maple syrup (optional)

Base
Mix ingredients together. Place in the bottom of a dish and pat down using your hands or a spatula. Slice banana circles and place onto the base.

Toffee
Mix all ingredients together until smooth. Pour over base and bananas.

Cream Topping
Blend all ingredients and pour on top of the toffee. Decorate your Banoffe Pie with dried or fresh banana rings and/or grated raw chocolate.

NOTE: *Store-bought oat groats are highly unlikely to be raw (they will have been steamed to clean and preserve them), but raw oat groats go rancid very quickly. As oats are a great health food (they are low in fat and high in various nutritious properties), they are a great ingredient to use if you are not hung up on being strictly raw.*

Green Tea Ice Cream
(Drew Hunt)

Prep: 20 minutes
Freeze: Refer to ice cream maker manufacturer's instructions

1 cup gunpowder green tea
3 cups water, boiling
1 cup honey
1 tablespoon vanilla
1 teaspoon sea salt
1 teaspoon puréed raw potato

Stir gunpowder green tea into boiling water. When tea returns to a boil take off flame and let sit until it reaches room temperature. Put into a nut bag or clean dish towel and squeeze the liquid out. Add ¼ cup of liquid (any leftover can be frozen for later or added to cold water to make iced green tea) to enough young coconuts (water and pulp) to yield 8 cups. Add honey, vanilla, sea salt, and puréed raw potato. Put into your ice cream maker and follow manufacturer's instructions.

This is delicious with grated raw chocolate and salt sprinkled on top. It is also very good with balled watermelon and honeydew. I also like mine mixed with the zest of several lemons or blood oranges. By far my favorite is a big bowl of blackberries and segmented blood oranges with scoops of Green Tea Ice Cream on top. With a glass of sparkling water, there is no better way to stay cool on a hot and humid day.

TESTIMONIALS

KEN ALAN

(Concierge and food & travel writer)

My Shetland Sheep Dog waited patiently for me at the top of the long driveway, wagging her tail in greeting as I finally made the final steps to the top. Out of breath, perspiring, and feeling a slight pull in my thigh muscles, I gave her a weak scratch behind the ears and looked back down the steep incline. At the bottom I noticed a figure moving briskly; a jogger who had taken my quiet lane as a little sojourn off the nearby trail. I watched the runner with envy, seeing the athleticism he possessed within that lean body; the carefree spirit in his strong strides. At the same time, I felt almost defeated. Time, disuse of muscles, and far too many rich meals had finally taken its toll on me. At 45, I felt overweight. I felt my age.

I serve as a concierge for a living, which means that when I set my mind to making something happen, *it is going to happen.* It was at that moment, panting next to my dog (who was hardly panting at all), I decided to dedicate my life to the Art of Balance—eating right, exercising, and practicing positivity.

Fast forward two years. I am now that whip-thin runner, approaching the long, steep hill with my Sheltie by my side. Together we lope easily up the incline to the top.

Commitment, dedication, and most of all, the love of life has helped me to become the physically fit and nutritionally balanced individual I had sought to be.

Here are some key points to the path I took in order to remain vital and ever-heading in the right direction.

Three Squares a Day: I make it a point to never miss a meal. I always keep a varied, though consistent diet that is as rich in super foods as possible.

98% Vegetarian: I rarely eat animal protein anymore. This is no easy feat considering I dine out for a living. Still, I find that unless there is a menu item that's important for me to taste and report on, I am able to keep my meat intake to its bare minimum. Best of all, I don't miss the stuff!

No Second Best for Me: I have a personal mandate which is, "Don't settle for second best." In the foods I shop for, and the restaurants I go to, I try to choose food purveyors offering the very best in quality. This doesn't mean I am forced to pay top dollar. As long as I keep my appetite in check, I am able to keep the dollars down by limiting portion sizes.

Water, Water Everywhere: It's all I drink. Okay, maybe I have a cup of tea or coffee every now and then, but I stay away from calorie-filled juices and I never consume soda.

Sweet Endings: Like most people, I usually crave something sweet at the end of my meal (especially after dinner). Instead of going for that cookie or piece of chocolate, I'll pop a couple raw cacao nips into my mouth. The bitterness immediately cuts my craving for sweetness, the deep richness sates my want for dark chocolate, and best of all, the cacao is actually really good for me.

There's Nothing Wrong with Cheating: Every once in a while, I'll splurge and eat something that's not so good for me. Denial, I've found, can ultimately be more detrimental in the long run.

Move! And Also, Mini-Move! Going back to running is the best activity I have ever done for myself. I'm fortunate that I am still able to maintain a steady stride for long distances without aches and pains. I have also adapted a stretching regime, always working on body parts to keep me limber while creating an ongoing tone.

Have a Lifestyle Buddy: Though I don't force my family to make the same lifestyle changes, I have subtly incorporated my methods into their daily lives, asking my wife and kids to try a particular food I'm preparing, go for a walk, or stop whatever we're all doing to do some stretching or breathing exercises. It is fun and cathartic at the same time.

Keep it Cool! A piece of advice I offer those who are making lifestyle changes is "Live it but don't bring attention to yourself," meaning, we'd all like support and praise from others ("Hey, you've lost weight!") but by continually telling others how many pounds you're taking off, or how hard you are training, it is a way to set oneself up to fail.

What Does the Future Hold? While I certainly can't predict how I'll be eating or feeling, for now I know that I feel way too good to deviate from this healthy lifestyle I have chosen for myself. Besides, my Sheltie wouldn't be able to forgive me if I couldn't make it up the hill again with her.

IRENE BOJCZUK

(www.returntocenter.com)

I've been on a personal growth, spiritual growth, and natural health path for at least the past 25 years. It has always made sense for me to choose the natural approach over any medical interventions whenever possible, and it also made complete sense for me to become a personal growth and success coach for a living.

I think it's common for people in my line of work to have had more than an average share of their own personal challenges, and that has certainly been true for me. The short list includes chronic seasonal depression and candida in my teens, twenties and into my early thirties; later bouts with severe chronic fatigue for several years; with a chronic and ever increasing set of symptoms such as intense body pain, hair loss, difficulty sleeping, and difficulty with focus and concentration. It was only in the past 4 years that I realized what I was dealing with was consistent with all the literature out there describing fibromyalgia.

My professional background geared me toward taking personal responsibility for my results and being ruthlessly determined to master my health just as much as any other goal. I was always searching out, studying, and trying on whatever I could find for healing my mind and body. I tried everything, including acupuncture, homeopathy, holistic medicine, macrobiotics, all sorts of natural supplements and even traditional medications to some degree. Everything I tried certainly moved me along on my path but nothing fully resolved the poor health that was under the surface in my life.

I was put in contact with a medical intuitive who told me, "Irene, I swear to you, if you do exactly what I tell you to do, you will heal completely." I decided to take him on and he proceeded to turn my diet around from everything I thought was right. Ultimately, he had me eating only raw fruits and raw salads with no oils and very little fats in the form of nuts and seeds. I eliminated all meat, dairy, eggs, grains, legumes, vinegars, oils, caffeine, and processed foods and stopped cooking food altogether. A few months into this I also did a 3-day water fast (taking in only water for 3 days, with rest) to speed up my healing. The results were so amazing that they far exceeded my greatest wish. I had signed on for this diet in hopes of eliminating the body pain. In that first 3-day fast, indeed all the pain did go away—to my utter amazement. I was not ready to believe it and assumed that the pain would probably return once I started eating again. But the truth is that about 95% of the pain was gone by the second day of fasting and it has remained so for the past 2+ years as long as I adhere strictly to the low fat raw vegan diet.

To tell the whole truth, I have struggled with cravings and missing the foods I used to enjoy. In the beginning, I tried to have the occasional treat, telling myself it would be harmless if I had a piece of fried chicken once a week. I actually found myself craving foods I had not even eaten in 25 years. And yes, sometimes I bought and ate an entire bag of potato chips. Eventually, in the early stages of this transition, I came to realize that I wasn't getting the results I had been promised because I wasn't adhering to the plan. It was only after I stopped cheating entirely for several months that I was able to experience the full benefits I'm reporting now. And even after that, I would sometimes find myself incapable of saying no to cooked or processed food that was within reach at a party or around my family. Fortunately and unfortunately, I got immediate feedback after eating those foods. Within a few hours at most I began to notice screaming pain returning in my neck or back. Each time I cheated, I was reminded of how critical it was for me to commit 100% to this program if I really wanted total health.

Now, in just over 2 years on this diet, I remain 95% pain free or better. I no longer find clumps of hair in my shower or sink drain—there is no hair loss anymore, and I can fall asleep with ease as long as I have had sufficient calories that day. People keep commenting on the quality of my skin and how I look overall. But beyond that, I have found a level of peace, a positive outlook, and the mental clarity and focus I never thought was possible.

The well-being that has become my normal state is far beyond anything I imagined possible for myself, and it far outweighs the social inconvenience of eating differently than my friends and family. I want to encourage anyone out there who is struggling with diminished health in any way to take on the challenge of stepping away from the mainstream approach to health.

Keep your eye on the prize—full health of mind, body, and emotions. The total picture is to have clear mental faculties, good memory, strong focus and concentration, energy and vitality, a pain-free enjoyable body, full mobility, emotional poise, a positive outlook, inner peace, creative inspirations, a spiritual connection that is strong at your core, great looking skin, and ideal weight. This has been my experience even at only 2+ years since starting, and I have not yet even fully mastered the fitness component.

SALLY BOWDLE

Growing up, I had endless mystery illnesses. I was the sick kid in class who no one wanted to sit next to. Like clockwork, every morning I just couldn't keep my breakfast down. This pattern continued on and off for years. It wasn't until my college years that the signs started to add up. Once, I collapsed from gas pains outside the dining hall after a standard meal of chicken fingers, fries, and soda. A few years later, a friend offered me a raw snack bar. I took one bite and was instantly nauseous. My solution to feel better was to eat something familiar— Goldfish® crackers and Kool-Aid®. I looked down at my orange and day-glo red snack and reflected on the nut, seed, and fruit bar that had supposedly made me ill. How could such a harmless food cause a reaction? Something about my unnatural snack showed me the pattern of how I had been eating—two decades of the standard American diet of highly processed foods. I knew something had to change.

For starters, I cut out my morning "weight gain shake" (it was just corn syrup and milk protein). No more waffles and bagels for breakfast and suddenly I was no longer trapped in the bathroom! After years of baffled doctors and endless medical bills, the light bulb was on. I saw that I could simply choose different foods and see an instant impact on my well-being. It was truly the most empowering moment in my life. Eat different, feel different. There was no sacrifice or denial, because I felt so much better!

What I want people to know is that this was not an overnight transformation. I feel a sense of compassion and patience is valuable throughout the process. It was 2001 when I decided to go dairy-free and gluten-free. I still struggled with mystery symptoms, illness, and weird rashes and it was a long process of alterations and eliminations; even to this day strange things come up.

The awakening continued with the realization that there was so much more to my transformation than food. At the time my life had room for serious improvement. I was working at a job that conflicted with my beliefs and I was in a relationship and living situation that wasn't supportive to my well-being. There was so much emotional healing and self love I needed to get to. Once I got to this understanding, the next steps started to fall into place.

It was 2009 when I finally had the courage to take the leap and quit my job. I was getting so inspired about cooking and baking gluten-free, I wanted to make a career out of it! I saw it was my life path to share with others what I had learned and help them along with their transformation. I completed the chef's training program at the Natural Gourmet Institute. I learned so much about different dietary choices, and was truly fulfilled to follow my dream.

Three years from graduation from chef school I find myself teaching others how to reawaken to healing foods, celebrating the possibility of wellness and wholeness. My work now is so diverse. I am thrilled to continue to learn every day.

My advice to seekers is to start small, start right now, and be bold in asking for help! Health foodies love to talk about food! Blessings on your journey.

JANET BUSHBY

My name is Janet Bushby and this is my amazing story after taking the Raw Challenge. I tried to lose weight all my life and sometimes it seemed to be working, but I was never satisfied with the amount of weight I lost or how long it took. I had 20 pounds left to get off when I started the Raw Challenge. The first week I lost 5 pounds, and I was so pleased.

When I decided to go raw I never expected to achieve this weight loss so fast. I also never expected to feel this great physically. I still have energy and don't feel like I am dieting but learning a whole new way of life. I'm happy and looking forward to the meals I prepare.

My diabetes is under control and I have been able to get off my medication for it. I am now working on getting off my blood pressure medication. My friends and relatives constantly compliment and congratulate me. They are happy for my achievements.

I don't only look healthier, I really am healthier! This has done wonders for me physically but I don't only want to talk about appearances. I am a much happier person and more confident person. When I lost the weight I started to feel better emotionally. I have confidence with my physical appearance and that makes me more out-going. I don't feel like I want to hide anymore.

I learned to adapt to what I am allowed to eat and what I like to eat. My likes and dislikes helped me to create wonderful recipes that I now share with others. I also received a ton of healthy and delicious recipes. I go to www. LivingDynamically.com and www.yummyplant.com for helpful tips and terrific new ideas. These websites have helped me tremendously, and I would like to suggest you visit them for new and useful plans to a healthier lifestyle.

The Raw Challenge has aided me in my search for a healthier, improved lifestyle and I am grateful for all the attention and help that was provided.

SHERYL CHAVARRIA

I have been on a natural healing path for the past 30 years after becoming a vegetarian at around age 20. Throughout my journey I have experienced a plethora of natural food lifestyles. Eventually my journey culminated in the raw foods arena which brought dramatic changes in my health, such as greater mental clarity, a huge increase of energy, clear skin, and a true glow of health. Soon thereafter, I was introduced to the importance of colon hydrotherapy which truly transformed my life. I then attended St. John's Academy in Maryland, became a Certified Colon Hydrotherapist, and opened a cleansing center.

To further my education, I attended Creative Health Institute (a well-known raw lifestyle, self healing facility, and educational center) where I became a Certified Health Practitioner and Educator, Raw Food Chef, Kitchen Director, and finally Director of the Institute. Shortly thereafter I opened a raw food café called Raw Can Roll Café to compliment the Wellness Center. I feel very blessed and thankful to have been given the opportunity to serve others.

LINDA COOPER

I grew up with, and later raised my children on, a standard American diet. I simply had not been educated to any alternatives, and I never had a reason to question our diets since everyone was relatively healthy.

That is, until my husband, Terry, was diagnosed with rheumatoid arthritis in 2005. Terry has always had a special talent for developing any side effects to pharmaceutical drugs. We knew that there had to be a better way to handle this diagnosis and then we heard about the "Hallelujah Diet" which practices 85% raw vegan to 15% cooked vegan. We decided to try the diet together, hoping to find a solution to Terry's illness.

The first few months were very, very hard. I fell into a bit of a depression once the magnitude of our decision hit me. Everything I had ever been taught and had ever known about food had been wrong. Just a trip to the grocery store became daunting. I began to question my ability to provide my family with truly nutritious food that actually tasted good. How have we been so misguided?

Determined to keep my family truly healthy, I submerged myself in raw cookbooks and joined a raw potluck and support group hosted by Lisa Montgomery.

Eventually, navigating through the organics aisle became easier, green juice became palatable, and most importantly, Terry was feeling better.

TIFFANY EDWARDS

When I heard about the Raw Challenge, at first I was hesitant, but I wasted no time signing up. I had just gotten over a bout of being sick and not being able to eat anything. I was done feeling like I couldn't help myself and felt that if anything the challenge could help.

When I started this, I didn't know where it would take me. I knew it would bring me to a healthier lifestyle, but I never thought it would have me examining myself and others and the food we place into our mouths. I always thought it would be difficult and that it would cost too much. Though it is a bit pricy to buy all organic, if you are on a budget like myself you need to make a compromise. Little by little I add things I need to my raw regimen. Raw honey one day, a bag of raw cashews the next. Coconut oil is my impulse buy one day, and a spiralizer the next. I don't stick with salads or bland foods, I branch out and make each meal interesting. If you want to be healthy and you feel weird about what you're doing, find comfort in it.

It came about that it was time for the Catholic tradition of Lent. I thought this was as good a time as any to start making a change, so I decided to cut out sugar, meat, dairy, and alcohol. I dropped 20 pounds over the course of two months. Then I hit my dreaded plateau of 180 pounds. I was running, walking, and doing 5Ks (3.1 miles) for the first time in my life. I felt good, but after returning from my diet I noticed more and more how food was affecting me. I would get headaches, feel sluggish, had no energy, and at 3 P.M. I would be falling asleep at my desk. I knew it wasn't right to feel this way, and then I came across the Raw Challenge. I thought, what could it hurt? Come to find out, it could only help me tremendously.

Each day I created something new, I started my day with smoothie and would build from there. I stepped on the scale on Friday morning and I had lost 6 pounds in 6 days! I was overjoyed. It amazed me that I was eating more, feeling full, but still maintaining a low fat and low-calorie diet.

I find myself listening to my body more; if I am hungry I eat. I love that I can cut up a watermelon and eat this all morning and afternoon and I need nothing more. After 14 days of eating 100% raw, I have dropped 9 pounds (almost 10)! I feel energized, and my body feels amazing! Though I may have occasions where I have meat, this challenge has opened my eyes to that which I have never known. It showed me that I didn't need certain things, that I could live without them and that my body benefited so very much from the challenge. Do it yourself, and do it *for* yourself. The most surprising thing to me was that each day someone would come up to me and tell me how awesome I looked, how skinny I was becoming, and how I was doing it. What a great and wonderful feeling!

SCOTT GRYZBEK

My mom, bless her soul, took very good care of our diets when I was growing up. Sugar, snack foods, sugary cereals—she wasn't having any of it. We hated it. But as I got older, I realized my mother had given me a tremendous gift, a foundation of health that would keep me strong through much travail.

Thankfully, my story of really finding health foods starts with that foundation, because I was no health foodist in college. Chicken wings and cheese steaks, beer and bad pizza. I went from a fit, ripped 135 pounds in high school to a flabby, soft 185 pound chunkster upon college graduation. I was in need of a change.

My path started shortly upon moving to Philadelphia after graduation. I came upon a health food store and was introduced to a world I had never seen before: gorgeous produce, all kinds of crazy cheeses (previously, our fancy cheese was the white American), chocolates, and so many brands I had never heard of. I was smitten. It wasn't really for health, but for the uniqueness, the difference from everything I had ever seen. I started to cook for myself and ate healthier, less processed meals. I found myself losing some weight and enjoying myself more.

In between jobs, I volunteered for an organic farm, and as a gift, they gave me a copy of *Nourishing Traditions,* by Sally Fallon. This was the first time I had heard something about diet that actually made sense. I quickly got rid of almost all the processed foods in my house, started fermenting raw vegetables, and grew all my food or got it from local farmers.

This change in attitude—the standpoint that if my ancestors didn't eat it or if I couldn't get it locally, I wouldn't eat it—made all the difference. Since I've been following this lifestyle (which includes a tremendous amount of raw and fermented vegetables and fruit as well as very local pasture-raised meat, milk, and eggs), my health has been tremendous, as has been my family's.

In the time since, I've been blessed to be able to start my own company, Zukay Live Foods, which is based on the tremendous health benefits of raw, fermented vegetables. I believe in my heart that our natural state is complete health, and Zukay is my way to give back to everyone to help them receive that health.

DREW HUNT

The first few days of the Raw Challenge were not easy. My jaw grew tired from the constant chewing. I was grazing constantly; apples, almonds, kale, and carrots. Nothing I ate gave me the satiated and full feeling I was used to and craved. I found it difficult to fall asleep at night. I was cranky and hungry. Yes, my mind became focused . . . on steak, cheese, bread, and gin. Fasting seemed easier than this middle path of eating only living raw organic fruits, vegetables, nuts, and seeds. I had very little hope of lasting the week without a few slices of thick buttered bread and a few martinis with those big oily, salty green olives.

But the third day's dawn greeted me, already awake, with a new outlook and motivation to go out for a swim. My energy became stronger, more constant, calmer, and more focused. I swam about a half mile that morning and ate melon, berries, dark chocolate, and carrot juice. If you can try very hard to eat 100% raw until about the fourth or fifth day you *will* begin to feel the effects. My body felt vital as soon as I woke. Prior to eating raw I struggled to wake in the morning. I would pull my achy body from bed, holding the railing while I hobbled down the steps to drink strong black coffee and take my pills. The fourth day I simply woke and easily and painlessly went downstairs for some water and fruit on my way to the YMCA for my swim. People started telling me I was glowing and the abundant energy put me in a delicious mood. I felt strong and confident and *good* for the first time in years. I was swimming a half mile in the morning and a half mile in the evening and tackling projects long overdue.

In the weeks that followed I underwent a drastic transformation. Every aspect of my life was affected. I purged my house of clutter and now live in the simplicity of less. I continued to swim daily and began some light core training. My posture greatly improved, my mind was rejuvenated and it felt like every cell in my body was vital and alive. Addictions lost their grip and my desire for fat, sugar, simple carbohydrates, coffee, and gin simply dissolved. For the first time in quite a long time hope—for many things I thought no longer possible—returned and I found myself living with presence in the moment.

I still do not own a dehydrator, juicer, or high-speed blender. I like to keep it simple and eat mostly nuts, seeds, fruits, and vegetables which I carry with me. I buy a fresh juice every day and make a smoothie many mornings. I did spend $30 on the little gizmo that makes zucchini noodles and enjoy a big bowl of my "I Can't Believe This Isn't Pasta" (see page 126) when I want a more traditional meal.

I continued eating 100% raw and lost 25 pounds. I stopped taking high blood pressure medication after 15 years. My asthma, arthritis, and fibromyalgia symptoms were greatly reduced. While having such surplus energy from eating 100% raw was very healing for me it also made me feel ungrounded. I now eat completely raw five days a week. Two days a week I also eat cooked vegetables, grains, and legumes. One meal a week I eat anything I desire, usually ending the week with a pint of Ben & Jerry's Karamel Sutra. I feel balanced.

It's hard in the beginning, but aside from quitting smoking and learning to properly and regularly practice meditation, I can think of nothing that has improved my health and life so much as a raw vegan diet. I wanted to share my experience and so I created the Kimberton Whole Food's Raw Food Challenge. I have co-conducted the challenge with Lisa Montgomery twice and I hope you will afford yourself the *metta* (Pali word for loving-kindness) to try at least one week of eating raw food. It very well may alter and ameliorate the course of your life.

DR. KAREN IZZI

When Lisa started the Raw Challenge, my friend Phyllis and I agreed that something needed to change in our lives. We were both turning 45 and were at our heaviest weights. We both work hard and play hard. Losing weight and getting a bit more fit seemed to be our biggest motivation to participate in the Raw Challenge. We began a week before it officially started in order to prepare ourselves mentally. It would be easier for me to make these dietary changes because for years I have been vegetarian, vegan, and even macrobiotic. Phyllis, on the other hand, was a junk-food junkie. Baby steps, for each of us. My thing was chips (salt) and hers, sugar, in any form.

Since we live in an imperfect world, there is no such thing as the perfect diet. However, after trying all of the latest fads, eating raw foods does not feel like a diet. It is real because the foods *are* real. It feels natural and wholesome because it *is* natural and wholesome. Consuming raw, whole foods is not only relied on for specific health concerns but for anyone who would like to properly cleanse, detoxify, and nourish their systems. If you are tired of feeling sluggish and forgetful without a reasonable excuse, then I encourage you to make small changes until your diet contains at least 60% raw foods, then 85%. For some, this will take a few months and a lot of will power, while for others it will mean smaller steps toward the many rewards. During the first few weeks of the transition your body will be going through a tremendous amount of cleansing as it adjusts to whole foods. The farther away you are from consuming an all raw diet, the more symptoms of cleansing you will notice. Without sugar, salt, and excess fat, the body will eliminate properly and may show signs like skin eruptions, headaches, fatigue, increased flatulence, and bad breath. For a few days you may feel as though you won't make it without coffee, a donut, or a beer but trust me, you will!

Going raw is like being put into someone else's body. For the first few weeks you may not recognize yourself, the new attitude, or the tremendous amount of new energy. Your clothes will fit more comfortably and you won't feel the need to suck in your stomach when you sit down. The taste of raw, organic foods has diminished frequent cravings for sweet/salt and dieting obstacles have disappeared because my body is being fully nourished. My energy levels are so terrific that I don't have any cravings for those "other foods." The changes in my body are hard to describe. The changes in my spiritual and emotional self are significant as well. The support of our friends in the Raw Challenge has been most important. We have shared food, snacks, and recipes. This challenge has been amazing and has changed my life forever.

ALLISON JEROME

My name is Allison. I am a 16-year-old in high school. I decided to do this challenge with my mom, not only to support her in our journey, but also to change my eating habits. This challenge seemed easy at first, but I was wrong. For the first couple of days it was easy for me. I had a fruit smoothie in the morning with an apple, then I would have a salad for lunch, and chicken with a garden salad for dinner. On the second day I had a headache. But it went by quick. From eating a ton of fruits and vegetables, I had a lot of energy. I was rarely tired during the day. At the end of the first week I lost 4 pounds! I was really happy about that! I kept up the good work for the second week and lost 3 pounds. When the challenge was over I was so glad: I had lost 7 pounds!

TAMMY JEROME

My name is Tammy. I am a 50-year-old woman, extremely overweight, and was told a week before the Raw Challenge that I am diabetic. The last 25 years have been spent juggling a full time job and a family. Now that I have a senior in college and a junior in high school, I have decided it's time to take some time for myself. When I heard about Lisa's Raw Challenge, I jumped at the chance to be a part of it. I figured it was a great way to learn something new and get a jump start on my weight loss. Throughout the Challenge, I kept a diary of my thoughts and feelings, which I will share for you here:

July 14, 2012
Here we go! Attended the first meeting this morning. I have never been so scared and overwhelmed! I feel like I have bit off more than I can chew, however I am determined to make changes. I am going to have to take this one day at a time and one meal at a time!

July 15, 2012

First full day. I weighed myself first thing this morning and despite what the scale said I am staying positive. For breakfast this morning I sliced an apple. Two hours later my stomach was growling! I drank a glass of water and had a banana. I do not feel bloated or weighed down with food. I don't feel hungry either. I do have a slight headache, but I think that's because I haven't had caffeine today.

July 18, 2012

Wow! I woke up before the alarm clock and felt really, really good! I can't tell you how long it has been since I woke up feeling refreshed! My skin definitely looks better. The circles under my eyes are fading and they don't seem as puffy! Maybe there is some truth to this good, clean living!

At the workshop, Lisa made the comment, "if you don't want to look at your stuff, don't go raw." There really is nowhere to hide when you don't have that bag of chips or that brownie to stand behind. Physically I feel good, but I have so much emotional baggage that I need to deal with.

July 24, 2012

Weighed myself this morning, I am down 8 pounds. I got on the scale and back on again to make sure it was accurate. Man does that add fuel to my fire! I can do this!

July 25, 2012

Have I mentioned how good I have been sleeping? I go to bed and fall asleep quickly and I am not tossing or turning and waking up every couple of hours. Before I started this challenge I would fall asleep on the couch almost daily. I had no energy and felt terrible all the time. Feeling good eating raw is definitely an incentive to stay with it.

July 28, 2012

Last official day of the challenge! I weighed myself this morning and have lost a total of 9 pounds! Going raw is not a diet, it is a lifestyle change. It takes commitment, determination, and will power just as anything in life does if you want to make a change for the better.

Since the challenge I have dropped from 100% raw to about 60% raw. I still feel good but not like I did at 100% raw. My plan is to continue the raw lifestyle and slowly increase it to 80% or 90%. At this point I am not convinced that I will ever do 100% raw, but never say never! I plan on moving forward one day at a time, one meal at a time, using baby steps . . . and a lot of determination.

LU ANN LIBERATORI

I stumbled into my raw food journey during my mom's illness and was investigating diet as an alternative to chemo treatments. As a carb/junk food addict I did not understand it much, but I wanted to try the raw food diet. I started very simply with green smoothies. I was told that my mom should be only drinking green smoothies at that point because she could not put anything in her stomach as the cancer had already spread to her stomach. We drank green smoothies but ate everything else.

I believe these smoothies had kept her alive for another year. Her cancer was very aggressive and rapidly moving at a high speed, but the green smoothie seemed to slow it down, almost to a halt. Her doctor said he was amazed how her cancer slowed. She proudly told him that I gave her green smoothies, and he told her to keep it up.

Unfortunately, my mom lost her battle with cancer after it had spread to her liver. After her transition, I decided to check into the raw food diet more thoroughly and found Lisa Montgomery.

Lisa's website had postings for raw potlucks and I thought about attending one. I was concerned about attending her potluck because I am deaf and felt it would be frustrating for me to make sure I understand what everyone is saying. I decided to bite the bullet and went to Lisa's potluck. I felt the patience of the group and Lisa welcomed me with open arms. I felt like a guardian angel led me to Lisa as she became my first teacher in the raw food lifestyle. I decided to intern at a raw food café near my home and learned a lot about the diet/lifestyle and felt very good.

One day I did my usual shopping at my local health food store and noticed that Lisa was having a Raw Challenge. I decided to take the challenge and slowly incorporate the raw food into my diet. During this challenge, I found out a lot about myself. One self-discovery was that I am a carb/junk food addict. When I am stressed I crave carbs and sugars. As a recovering addict, I needed to find something else to eat or do when I am stressed. I needed to change the phrase raw food "diet" into raw food "lifestyle." "Diet" is such a negative term for me, but "lifestyle" is more positive. I knew I needed to incorporate living foods into my lifestyle and went about it slowly. To do this slowly, I switched my mindset to recognize that following a living food lifestyle is not a burden but rather a blessing and is vital for my physical, mental/emotional, and spiritual health.

I also needed to change my mindset that I am not living to eat, but eating to live. As of now, I drink smoothies in the morning and my one big meal for the day is mostly raw. Slowly and steadily I am climbing back on the raw food wagon, and I will take one day at a time with the living food lifestyle.

DAWN LIGHT

I love a challenge, so when Lisa decided to have her Raw Challenge, I was psyched! Sharing a journey with like-minded people toward a common goal is fun and inspiring. I knew I would be more likely to stay committed when there were other people who expected me to do the best I could do, and report back on what I had actually done. For me, that was a great way to share this particular journey.

We kicked off the Challenge by having our first meeting in a great space above the Kimberton Whole Foods store. Lisa began by teaching us how to get started with raw foods. She covered some favorites such as wheat grass juice, watermelon juice, nut milk, and smoothies. We also discussed raw food basics, which are simpler than most people expect. Who knew preparing and eating raw foods could be so easy, energizing, and yummy? Lisa made learning fun, interesting and engaging. We all left the gathering feeling motivated and ready to see what we could achieve when we incorporate more raw foods into our diets.

I really liked the way Lisa planned the Challenge, too. The kick-off, regular gatherings, follow-up emails, Facebook group, and potlucks kept us engaged and committed. We shared our progress, insights, challenges, and tips . . . all of which I found helpful and rewarding.

The gatherings kept us all on track because we had given our word that we would do our best. We cared about each other and the progress we made. Everyone's journey was unique, so I learned many things from the others involved. We were all inspired by everyone's story about what brought them to the raw food lifestyle and the changes they wanted to experience in their lives through it.

When I was growing up my mother was always trying new ways to make us healthier. I remember her regularly doing seven-day apple fasts. I think we did our first family cleanse when I was 11. We used something I remember being called "deterg" that I know now had psyllium husks in it. She raised us on a whole-food diet with healthy alternatives like Tiger's Milk. Even though I was never really sick, other than the occasional cold or flu, I felt a need to be as healthy as I could be.

My first introduction to the raw food diet was in 2000. I was in the

Kimberton Whole Foods store, hugely pregnant with my second daughter, when I met a woman who was planning a raw food class. I took her class on how to prepare an entire raw food meal. The culmination was our consumption of the meal, including dessert. It was blissful. And after filling myself with wholesome, nutritious, and delicious raw food, my body wasn't going to settle for anything less.

My diet has evolved since then. For me, on any given day, I eat from 75% to 100% raw. I do what I can within my schedule and what I have available, knowing that the more I plan ahead, the easier it is to stay raw. I pay attention to how I feel after I eat. This helps me stay away from what isn't good for me, and helps me eat what is good for me. That's one of the advantages of eating raw foods: I know when I've given my body what it needs because I feel great!

During the Raw Challenge I learned that friendship and camaraderie are nourishing and make food taste better. We spent one entire gathering preparing sauerkraut. Lisa taught us the basics. Then we chopped, sliced, and spiralized veggies while talking about our challenges, successes, and discoveries. It was a bonding experience that put good energy into our food and our bodies.

KRIS SCHAFFER
(Nutrition Coach, raw foodie, and kale enthusiast)

When I began my two-week Raw Challenge, my goals were to increase my energy level, clear my skin, initiate better digestion, and maintain optimal health. This journey, as I knew with any habit change, would be difficult. Some of my initial concerns were whether I would be satisfied with just eating raw foods, and if I would need to make additional time to prepare these foods. Given my fast metabolism, I also had concerns about losing weight.

For the first few days, I was quite lazy and prepared simple shakes which contained kale and fresh fruit (watermelon, cherries, blueberries, mango, banana, and cantaloupe) with Garden of Life raw meal protein blended with coconut or almond milk. As you can imagine, it got quite boring after a few days. I then incorporated mixed green salads with raw nuts and veggies from my garden. For the first couple of days I felt extremely gassy. This feeling subsided as my digestive system soon adjusted to the additional fiber. I soon began incorporating beans and seeds for added flavor and protein. On the third and fourth day, I felt a greater sense of energy in the afternoons and my skin was starting to reflect a healthier glow. Also, with the increased fiber I felt fuller longer.

I decided to borrow my Mom's dehydrator and made some kale, zucchini, and baby bella mushrooms chips with fresh garlic, Himalayan salt, fresh cilantro, and cold-pressed sesame oil. Wow, what a fantastic snack to munch on in between meals. I've always had a liking for sunflower seeds and loved the mock tuna salad by Awesome Foods™. I decided to make my own version by soaking sunflower seeds overnight and combining fresh lemon juice, raw cashews, chopped scallions, mustard powder, and chopped celery. I thoroughly enjoyed my mock salad, which increased my motivational level. As the days passed, I continued to feel lighter and felt my eyesight had improved.

At week's end, I attended a potluck dinner at a friend's house and prepared a tasty green soup with cucumbers, avocado, green onions, and a handful of fresh basil and cilantro, with a hint of raw agave nectar. I also prepared a kale salad with red and green peppers, grape tomatoes, and beet greens covered with a white miso, raw tahini, and ginger dressing. Yummy! That night I weighed myself and to my amazement had gained two pounds!

My second week was a bit of an emotional setback. I developed oral candida which required me to eliminate all fruits, raw cashews, all sugars, carrots, beets, peas, and some cocoa products. I felt disappointed that I had come this far and now had to adjust my raw food choices to reduce my yeast overgrowth. I began consuming fermented foods and foods rich in probiotics such as kefir, yogurt, sauerkraut, and kombucha. I continued to incorporate my fresh green salads with selected fresh vegetables. As my intestinal flora restores itself, I will return to my truly raw diet.

I was eager to share my raw food experience with my mother after my first week. She was very supportive and excited for my beneficial results. She is my trusted mentor and my greatest inspiration for living healthy. With that said, I have shared with you her favorite Mixed Green Salad (see page 113).

MARY SCHAFFER

I've been eating raw foods ever since I can remember. I grew up in the mountains of northern Pennsylvania near Pottsville during the depression. My six siblings and I would venture into the woods and pick huckleberries, raspberries, blueberries, and teaberries. We would also collect tree twigs and branches from the woods and make homemade birch beer. We grew as many vegetables as we could fit into our backyard garden, from green beans to pumpkins. I still remember eating corn right off the stalk and inviting my friends from our neighborhood to enjoy one of our raw sweet potato parties.

Until just a few years ago, I had the luxury of unlimited gardening space, and I used it to my full advantage in growing herbs, vegetables, and small fruit trees in abundance. I utilized as much of the fresh produce as possible and either froze, canned, or stored the rest in my cellar. I started apricot trees from fruit pits, I dried hot peppers, and I canned countless jars of fresh tomatoes and homemade fruit jellies.

Now after raising my four children, and currently living in a small townhouse, I utilize my patio deck and my flower beds to grow herbs, tomatoes, and sweet peppers. In addition to my home-grown food, I also shop at local orchards and farms to prepare my daily raw food meals.

One of my favorite ways of preparing fruits and veggies is to process them in my juicer for a refreshing healthy drink. I try to re-purpose the pulp when I juice my organic apples and carrots and have shared two of my favorite recipes (see pages 178 and 110).

DAVE SCULLY

I grew up in a family that overall ate pretty healthy. A lot of our meals were made by my mother and were of fresh ingredients. We still ate the standard American diet (SAD) but with a little more emphasis on fruits and vegetables. One of my favorite snacks as a kid was either a bowl of frozen peas or frozen blueberries.

My first introduction to eating a different type of healthy foods came from my uncle Grant who my brothers and I thought of as our weird and crazy uncle from California. There were various reason why we thought he was weird, but among of them was his strange diet. When Uncle Grant would visit he would show up with strange, exotic foods like pomegranates, star fruit, kiwis, and passion fruit—foods I had no idea even existed. He introduced us to crazy things like drinking green smoothies, wheatgrass, and staying away from fast food, sodas, sugar, and too much dairy and breads. Growing up mostly in South Dakota there wasn't a lot of exposure to other ways of eating. Meat was for protein. Milk and dairy were for healthy bones and the rest was because it was good for you. I had a few friends who were vegetarian but, like my uncle, they were weird.

Then one year I went to work for my uncle and lived with his family. Everything about the way I ate changed. There was very little meat and when there was it was wild caught or grass fed with no hormones or antibiotics. Dairy was nonexistent except for a little bit of goat cheese here and there. I got used to eating raw granola instead of sugary cereal for breakfast with fresh fruit and fresh apple or orange juice in place of milk. I ate more vegetables and fruit, was introduced to gluten-free products, and started eating avocados as a snack. There was even the famous Grantwich: a sandwich made of Ezekiel® bread, avocado,

Brussels sprouts, tomato, and some goat cheese. It was great! I felt great, slept better, and my skin cleared up. I didn't have energy crashes in the middle of the day or after I ate lunch. I felt stronger in all areas of my life. I was hooked and wanted to know more, learn more.

All of this ended up having a major impact on the course of my life and a strong influence on my choice of career. Jump forward many years and I am now a Practitioner of Oriental Medicine who emphasizes food as medicine. I tell all my patients that in any tradition food is considered the highest form of medicine. And the journey continues.

BARBARA SHEVKUM, RAWFULLY TEMPTING

(www.rawfullytempting.com)

My adventure into raw food began in October, 2009. Surprisingly, I discovered joy in the most unexpected place. What started as an exploration into healing resulted in a whole new toolbox for creating food that is literally alive with color, texture, flavor, healing nutrients and life! I quickly fell in love with a whole new palette of ingredients . . . and a new palate for tasting them.

Raw is beautiful. It's alive . . . and it offers me an incredible challenge to create new and exciting textures that are decadent, delicious, and nutritious. And the best is, I'm eating food that is chock full of healing properties, the way nature intended. Uncooked food from nature comes with its own enzymes, which means the body does not have to work as hard to digest it. If you are chronically ill, this enables your body to conserve some of its resources that can be used toward healing.

I am not 100 percent raw, however. My personal choice in my personal space is raw, and I can say with all of my heart that I feel much better when I eat mostly raw, and for that reason, I try to incorporate as much of that as I can.

I write about raw food. I teach how to prepare raw food, and I love the fact that raw food can have such a positive impact on my health. I came from the corporate world, and sickness took me out of it. I have no desire to go back, and am trying to take all that I've learned and move forward in the world, doing what I love to do.

For those with health issues, I do emphasize caution when branching off on your own and do not advise ignoring your physician unless you understand the risks involved. I know that those of us suffering with chronic illness want so much to heal, that we gravitate toward people pronouncing they've "healed it all." Each of us is unique, and the path to healing is not a cookie cutter process. My goal is not to dissuade anyone from trying this to get well, but to have you err on the side of caution. Small steps forward are a lot better than large steps backward.

I'm a raw vegan chef and I create recipes that help others transition to a healthy and fun way of eating and living. Just because I post decadent desserts, does not mean I live off them. I'm not much different than a pastry chef, who creates stunning (albeit unhealthy) treats that others enjoy, but rarely is tempted to eat food that he or she works with every single day. Give me a huge salad in my big stainless steel bowl, and I'm happy. Undoing old habits takes time, and commitment. The key is to not beat yourself up, but to take notice. Pay attention and be clear at what you want to accomplish. Learning to be kind to yourself and admit that you are worth the effort seems to be a common thread for many of us.

PHYLLIS TERRY

At my last doctor visit my overall cholesterol level was 253 and I refused to start taking cholesterol medicine because of the known side effects. My doctor made a deal with me that I had to lose 30 pounds by December 2012, and my cholesterol level had to be 200 or lower or I would have to go on medication for six weeks. I agreed to this deal knowing that if I started eating better and exercised, then I would lose the weight and bring down the high cholesterol level.

A few weeks later my partner, Karen, told me that Lisa Montgomery was hosting a Raw Challenge and that it would be a great way for me to lose weight and start feeling better. I was a bit reluctant at first to try it since I love meat and cooked food and didn't think I would last on this type of diet or lifestyle. I thought about it and agreed to do it. The week prior to the challenge I mentally prepared myself by cutting back on meat.

At the first week's meeting I sat in the back of the room and listened as everyone introduced themselves and told us what they wanted to achieve from this challenge. I found that there were a lot of people in the group like myself who wanted to incorporate raw into their diet.

During the first week of the challenge I had several deadlines at work and I thought to myself, "How am I going to get through this with my stress level increasing each day and no comfort food?" During that week I was surprisingly able to stick to the raw plan and my cravings for sweets and chips went away. I decided to weigh myself at the end of the first week and to my surprise I had lost 6 pounds.

During week two, I decided to get sushi from my local grocery store and finally decided on tuna sashimi which is completely raw and something I had never tried before. I also decided to get one of the store's sparkling juices which I knew had sugar but remembered it not being very sweet. I finished my sashimi and started drinking the sparkling juice, only to find that it was too sweet for me. Karen told me that my body was cleansing itself and that by doing that my tastes would change, which they definitely did. I never liked seltzer water but found that it was the only carbonated drink I could tolerate. I did feel better but I started to miss cooked foods and meat.

The second week was much like the first week. I found I had more energy at work as my water consumption increased with eating raw and I noticed that

I wasn't eating as much as the first week. One night I did go out to dinner at a Vietnamese restaurant and had a chicken and rice meal which filled me up but not to the point where I was uncomfortable. I remembered a time when I would have that same meal but still be hungry afterward. That Thursday I weighed myself again and found that I had gained a pound back from the six I had lost. However, I was okay with that because I knew it may have just been an off day. We weren't able to make it to the final Challenge meeting, but Karen and I decided that we would continue this journey together. I weighed myself again in the last week and I had lost the pound I gained the previous week.

I don't think I would have been able to accomplish any of this had it not been for the group's support at the meetings and Karen's support at home. Had it not been for her creative non-cooking, I wouldn't have lasted two days before falling back on my old bad habits.

I find that I am sleeping better and not snoring as much as I used to and my energy level has increased. I have been told by quite a few people that I am "glowing" and my skin looks great. I have also lost my double chin and my stomach does not stick out as much as it used to. This was a great experience and I would tell anyone who is interested to definitely try it, even if raw does not become a lifestyle you pursue. Thank you, Lisa, for providing me with the tools to accomplish this goal.

ROBERT CHARLES WHITE, PH.D.

At 43 years old, I was diagnosed with type 2 diabetes I did a lot of research regarding diets for type 2 diabetes and continued to monitor my blood glucose levels while beginning a daily exercise regimen. I learned about the raw food diet several years prior. When I was looking at what foods had positive effects and neutral effects on my blood glucose levels, it was clear that a raw diet may be ideal for me.

I signed up for Lisa Montgomery's Raw Challenge. Through my research prior to beginning the challenge, I learned that raw diets consist of a minimum of 75% raw food. I quickly calculated the food I had been eating over the past two days and realized I was already eating about 65% raw food, without even trying! As you can imagine, clearing the 75% hurdle was not difficult for me.

I attended a raw food lecture and cooking demonstration by world famous chef Cherie Soria of Living Light Culinary Institute and purchased a copy of her book, *The Raw Food Revolution Diet*. I patronized health food stores and read everything about raw food that I could get my hands on. I purchased a Vitamix® high-speed blender, a dehydrator, and a spiralizer, which have become an integral part of my diet. I also attended raw potlucks with some new friends from the Raw Challenge.

In 3 months, have I lost a total of 35 pounds. During this time, my insulin has decreased from 18 units daily to 10 units daily, then incrementally decreased to 8 units, then 6 units, then 4 units, then 2 units, then ZERO units daily. I am looking forward to my next appointment with my endocrinologist and my primary care physician, as I'm hoping to hear that I will be able to discontinue my oral type 2 diabetes medication as well. I attribute my success to educating myself about type 2 diabetes, eating a healthy diet consisting of a minimum of 75% raw food, and engaging in daily vigorous exercise.

FINAL WORDS

Congratulations! You've made it to the Finish Line of your Raw Challenge! You picked up the gauntlet and started the process of transforming your life and living to the fullest. The Raw Challenge has now come to a close, but in life the "finish line" continues to move as we grow and evolve emotionally, spiritually, and physically. One of the greatest gifts the raw lifestyle gives as you go through the challenges of life is a body and soul that supports you.

You need your body to be strong in order to deal with the highs and lows of life that are beyond your control. Once you heal your body physically you can work on the emotional and spiritual challenges so when the "stuff" of life comes your way, you are helping yourself stay on track.

My body is strong because I give it good fuel. Last year I broke my leg. Five pins, screws, and a plate later, I had a cast on and was on crutches. Because of the way I eat and live, along with my can-do attitude, the physical therapists were amazed at my progress. Attitude is everything and for me living this healthy lifestyle keeps me positive.

My challenge to you with this Raw Challenge is to make the commitment today that you are worth it as, one step at a time and one mouthful at a time, you begin to transform your life. You can do it. How do I know you can do it? Because I did it, and after almost 20 years, I am still doing it and I would never go back to the way I used to eat or live. The Raw Challengers stepped up and transformed their lives as detailed in this book. I challenge you to start today, and start living your life to its absolute fullest.

This is only the beginning of your transformation. Take some time to evaluate where you started, and consider where you would like to go. Make a list of your goals and objectives, and how you plan to reach them. If you don't set goals you won't ever achieve them. This is only the beginning of your true, healthy life. Again, congratulations on taking the all-important first step in your quest to "Live Dynamically!"

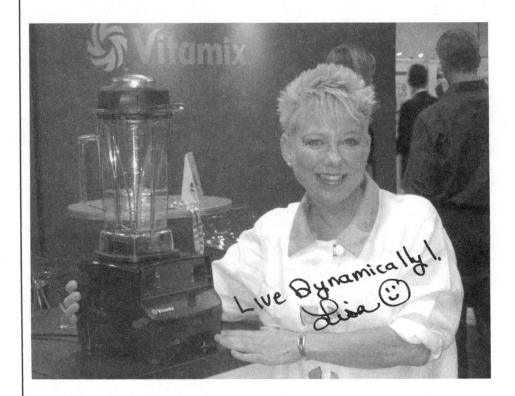

RESOURCES

Books

Cultured, Make Healthy Fermented Foods at Home—70+ recipes contributed by the world's leading natural health experts, edited by Kevin Gianni.

Wild Fermentation, by Sandor Ellix Katz

The Joy of Pickling, by Linda Ziedrich. This book requires some adjustments if you are leading a raw lifestyle (like omitting sugar in the recipes), but you can adapt the recipes and make them healthy.

Nourishing Traditions, by Sally Fallon. I reference this book for fermented and pickled foods. Again, you can adapt it to a raw lifestyle.

Food in Jars, by Marisa McClellan. This book is about preserving in small batches year-round. I use these recipes and adapt them for my needs by omitting sugar and using my own homemade juices in place of condensed juice.

Wheatgrass, Nature's Finest Medicine, by Steve Meyerowitz, Sproutman. This is an excellent resource to answer everything you wanted to know about wheatgrass and how to grow it.

Home Sweet, Home Grown: How to Grow, Make and Store Food, No Matter Where You Live, by Robyn Jasko.

The Body Ecology Diet, by Donna Gates. This is the first "healthy" book I bought when I first changed my diet after I found out I had food allergies and candida. This was a great book to get me started on a healthier way of life. It was recommended by my homeopath at that time. My diet has changed since then as it continues to change and grow as I do. Some of Donna's fermented recipes are also in *Cultured,* by Kevin Gianni, as mentioned above.

The Art of Fermentation, by Sandor Ellix Katz. This is an in-depth exploration of essential concepts and processes from around the world.

Designing with Natives, by John Rogers. A road map for backyard design and stewardship using native plants.

MAGAZINES

Urban Farmer: Sustainable City Living. This is of my all-time favorite magazines. They show you how to be a farmer in suburbia or in town. They also have great recipes. I love it, love it, love it.

Whole Living: Body + Soul in Balance

Mother Earth News: The Original Guide to Living Wisely

Energy Times: Enhancing Your Vitality Through Nutrition, Health & Harmony. This is a free magazine that you can find at your local healthy market or pharmacy. I look forward to reading this each month as it is full of helpful tips, facts, and recipes.

Alternative Medicine: Happy. Healthy. Holistic.

Eating Well: Where Good Taste Meets Good Health

Permaculture: Inspiration for Sustainable Living

Backwoods Home Magazine: Practical Ideas for Self-Reliant Living

WEBSITES

Ani Phyo: Eco-Stylist & Organic Food Author (www.aniphyo.com)

lalaraw: Vegan Raw Food Lifestyle, Recipes, and Health Tips (www.lalaraw.com)

Living Light: Making Healthy Living Delicious! (www.rawfoodchef.com)

Fully Raw (www.fullyraw.com)

Rawfully Organic Co-Op (www.rawfullyorganic.com)

Raw High Life (www.rawhighlife.com)

RECIPE INDEX

NOTES

NOTES

NOTES

NOTES

NOTES

NOTES

NOTES

NOTES

NOTES

NOTES